Workaholic

An Easy Guide to Help Moderate
Your Addiction

*(How to Break Work Addiction and Learn to Enjoy
Family and Life)*

Gregg Ledford

Published By **Phil Dawson**

Gregg Ledford

All Rights Reserved

Workaholic: An Easy Guide to Help Moderate Your Addiction (How to Break Work Addiction and Learn to Enjoy Family and Life)

ISBN   978-1-77485-741-0

No part of this guidebook shall be reproduced in any form without permission in writing from the publisher except in the case of brief quotations embodied in critical articles or reviews.

Legal & Disclaimer

The information contained in this ebook is not designed to replace or take the place of any form of medicine or professional medical advice. The information in this ebook has been provided for educational & entertainment purposes only.

The information contained in this book has been compiled from sources deemed reliable, and it is accurate to the best of the Author's knowledge; however, the Author cannot guarantee its accuracy and validity and cannot be held liable for any errors or omissions. Changes are periodically made to this book. You must consult your doctor or get professional medical advice before using any of the suggested remedies, techniques, or information in this book.

Upon using the information contained in this book, you agree to hold harmless the Author from and against any damages, costs, and expenses, including any legal fees potentially resulting from the application of any of the information provided by this guide. This disclaimer applies to any damages or injury caused by the use and application, whether directly or indirectly, of any advice or information presented, whether for breach of contract, tort, negligence, personal injury, criminal intent, or under any other cause of action.

You agree to accept all risks of using the information presented inside this book. You need to consult a professional medical practitioner in order to ensure you are both able and healthy enough to participate in this program.

Table Of Contents

Introduction

You are at the first chapter of our writing-word journey. Perhaps this is your first time you've come across me and you're looking forward to change in your world. Maybe you've already met me through my personal or professional circle, and you're looking forward to a change in your life. Whatever the case we would like to say welcome to the pages!

I've been told by a few individuals about the fact that "there is no work-life balance." It's a element of our lives, and we'll never be in sync every aspect of your life. There are movements which use terms such as work-life harmony and work-life integration and so on. They all aim to serve by providing more synergy and Zen joy and fulfillment, as well as less confusion, conflict, burnout and stress. While we may be working towards a more accepting view of the final game in harmony and harmony during those final dark times of the week when you're exhausted of it, I'm curious about what you're looking up or talking to yourself the most. The term "work lifestyle balance" is a common phrase regardless of whether you believe the word or not. regardless of whether you're looking for harmony, integration, balance or any other. This pathseeking to achieve work-life equilibrium -- is an inspiring challenge and will push you to get the things you desire by taking one step at a time while you read these pages.

In terms of "unapologetic," my wish is that you quit apologizing in your the workplace and at homesimply because you're living an agenda or are seeking a happier life. I know that you show respect to others both at work and home by asking permission. You may also be seeking forgiveness even when granted permission. Yet you came to this world with hopes aspirations, desires, and missions that are yours. It's time to look within take a deep look at your personal story is and stand up for something with no regret.

If you are familiar with you or not, here's some information about my background and the services I have to offer in these pages. I was a warrior in the corporate world and am now engaged to an executive and I am now a coach for corporate warriors. I've been commissioned to serve willing warriors by coaching them to improve their awareness, manage their anxiety and assist in making powerful decisions to lead a balanced life that they enjoy. I was compelled to leave my job in the corporate world to become coach, so that you do not have to quit yours. I am still stressed and can be overwhelmed at times. I too am one of the clients of my own process. This book is a compilation of my experiences from both inside and outside of the workplace through my interactions with others, as well as from personal experiences. I've put these lessons together to help you gain insights and techniques to overcome any stress and lead a more fulfilling life.

I would like to see that as you read this article, it feels like you're drinking a glass of wine with me, and you are talking about these examples and tools. This is an invitation to an exchange of ideas that will benefit you. You'll be equipped to sail through turbulent waters and experience effortless sailing, regardless of the length or how brief it runs.

At the moment I am able to provide coaching services to some companies. This is very satisfying when the work produces relationships, trust, loyalty and improvements over time. But, at the at the same time, I am aware that my reach is narrow, rather than broad and I am aware that my impact could be less than it should be. This book assists me in helping many more people with an extensive compilation of "Janine-isms" and the wisdom I impart with my clients, and which I've learned from other people encountered along the way. It is possible that you've heard of concepts similar to those in this book previously -either in books on leadership as well as self-help publications as well as through coaching, or from reading about how to apply the Law of Attraction. The goal of this book is to draw these concepts and other ideas together, and offer my personal viewpoint and this book is a compilation of the lessons I've employed for myself and have used with clients for more than 10 years.

As a personal note I'm honored to keep a part of me displayed on the shelf of my family, children, clients and friends to enjoy even after I've gone. I've always had a dream for all the time I remember being an author who was published. I thought it was necessary for me to write an instructional manual, guide or compass to document the time that I was in when I was at the forefront of leadership that was servant-hearted and able to assist the most people I could. The book I imagined myself writing would not just a glimpse into my world , but also a benefit to my clients. In it, I'd facilitate a dialogue between myself and the ideal client -- a writing coaching session that would draw out the fears and struggles my clients frequently face and motivate clients to lead their most fulfilling life. In my opinion I'm on the similar journey as you. Once you've found out something about me, what's the reason that's directing you to live the best life you can? Let's get the book out and begin our journey together.

Chapter 1: Mirror

The familiar, but not pleasant sound of alarm sounds on your phone. Is it already Monday morning It's Monday morning! The weekend flew by far too fast. What was the weekend like? You were working the majority of the time at catching up on emails and preparing your presentation for the next board meeting. At least, you weren't working in the office.

You're feeling a bit regret for not completing the exercise you made with your buddy. It was the time you wanted to started on a fitness program. But, it's not over, there's always the next weekend.

The list! Where is it? It's on the bedside table where you've woken up several times throughout your night, trying to recall all the things you have to accomplish this week. It's impossible to believe that it's so long and is very similar to the last week's checklist yet it must be completed.

The routine for the morning is one that's full. Eat breakfast, feed your children, and pack lunches (theirs and not mine ... it's yours if you can eat at work when you eat lunch even at all). Everyone is clean and tidy however the majority of the laundry is lying in piles. It is your responsibility to handle everything on your own, which is why you aren't tempted to employ a helper.

The children are taken to school the next morning, and your commute starts. You make a call during your commute to cut down on time. Bluetooth is enabled (safety first) This means you're free of hands while driving as a crazy individual and navigating the lane of corporate warriors who are heading to work.

The meeting goes well However, the deck that you've spent the weekend working on should be redesigned. It's a frequent theme in your own world. You wonder why there's always enough time to re-do it, but not enough time to finish it right in the first attempt?

In a flash you're at work. You search for the typical locations to park, lock up and walk in. A phone call arrives. You pick it up even though you realize that you're technically double-booked from as soon as you sit in your office. There's an emergency meeting scheduled to start at 4:45 p.m. Aren't you supposed to be leaving early for gymnastics double-practice this evening? Perhaps you'll be able to participate by telephone during your commute or perhaps you'll request your friend to join you in a carpool regardless of when it's your turn.

The clock is it's 9 a.m. on a Monday morning, and it's like you've lived nine times already.

Time. Friends or foes? In these days, there not enough. You're constantly looking forward to an extra hour during the day to finish the task or perhaps to be completely still. The task of completing your list of things to do efficiently is essential to you. What are we talking about ... You really are a perfectionist. Your work is the focus and it can be a source of satisfaction for you. But what is the price?

Today, it's normal to take working hours for longer, no matter if you're arriving earlier or staying longer. What do you complete the task? The work won't be done by itself. Sure, you have a team, but they are all buried as well, and you are the kind of jump-in-and-get-your-hands-dirty type that keeps everyone and everything afloat.

In the home, however the battle is real. The list of tasks is equally long and never completed at the time of day. Weekends are great for to catch up, but you believe that having a few extra time during the week would simplify things. You believe there's got to be some bright light at the end the tunnel. Perhaps you'll tick off a few items on your list of home projects when you reach that deadline at work.

Have you ever thought"Once this is over I'll breathe again. There will be some breathing room following this board's meeting and after the presentation, and after this deadline. There's always something else to sneak into. You'll throw your entire life into this project and all of the other aspects of your day feels like a mess.

We're back. Working hard and at a loss everywhere else. It's getting old! You're on the edge of burning out without a real parachute. Your work is extremely significant to you. It's not just an integral aspect of your life and your livelihood, but it also is also a source of income and benefits. It's been a long time since you've had to work and have come a long way to make a mistake right now.

The dedication to your work is admirable, however it's costing your peace and joy in other aspects that you live in. Perhaps all of them! On certain days, it seems as if you're about to take an airplane to an island far away and throw everything electronic from the boat and in the ocean when you arrive and never looking at it again.

Let's examine the various pieces to your thriving life. There's work to be done (we've shown that all well). Do you find it enjoyable for you? What is your level of satisfaction every day? While you may spend 8 hours (at the minimum, but it's actually more than that, like 11.) working every day There's more to you being an active human being with many aspects, much like a precious jewel.

We'll take a deeper review of each of these aspects soon However, for now, think of the following areas: money, career and health, relationships/significant others as well as recreation and fun families friends, friendships, support system, personal growth, physical environment, Self-care, Higher Power/Higher Self. I'm betting that one or more of these areas are struggling without your notice currently. This isn't the time to be judging yourself for this, but instead to simply be aware of your own reality (even when it's ugly).

This is among the first tests I conduct with my clients as we coach together. There are often tears, either out of the shock of the simple validation of what they knew. If you look at the satisfaction or lack of it, in every aspect of your existence, then you may not need to consider your conclusions. However, now that they're there ... you'll find that it's hard to ignore them. It's like the ultimate rubbernecking with damaged pieces of yourself throughout your surroundings.

If any of these seems familiar this book is the one for you at this time within your journey. What a blessing to find this common ache mirroring itself at exactly the time that you need it? In this article, I'll guide you on a journey that will aid you in taking your life back one minute at a moment, so that you are able to get your groove back at work, life, and wherever you like.

Chapter 2: Revolution

Sometimes, you'll encounter an event that opens a new path for you didn't anticipate or plan for. It's a kind of revolution. This chapter will share with you about my personal corporate journey and the gradual burn which eventually led to burning out, and the moment that changed everything , and made me cry.

A few years ago, I graduated from college with an associate's education in the field of food sciences. I ended up in an internal research and development position in Mars, Incorporated. I was doing what I believed was my true calling, however, I was apprehensive about an experience that was different. I was able to move around in different jobs until I ended up in the department of human resources, which was where I was in charge of procedures for managing talent, including appraisals and development planning as well as succession planning. In this capacity, where I learned about executive coaching. We'd coach our managers to support them in their development.

Executive coaches possess a strong presence and a tough-love method of looking up at their clients' faces, to assist them in determining what they need to alter within their work environment. They are able to uncover a client's growth goals, and the goals of their bosses, colleagues, or the entire team. While watching the coaches and began to understand their style and the impact of their actions, I noticed that their actions resonated with me.

In the beginning, I'd never had coaching experience, and I'd never played as a coach. However, I felt a strong pull towards their presence and their teachings. I was looking for a greater and more profound understanding of me. I wanted to make a connection to myself, one that ties the person I am both inside and outside of the office. In addition, I wanted to be the person who could achieve the goals I had set for myself and not those that I had created through an online survey that gave feedback to 360 people. Perhaps you have a connection to this yearning for something different or more. Maybe you're seeking clarity on what you want or the best way to achieve it.

I was attracted by the idea of becoming a coach. I would like to be the spark that brought on the lightbulbs of others or helped them shine brighter. The seed was planted deep inside the inside of me, an "someday perhaps" idea that was tucked within the potter's shed for the spring cleaning of our greenhouse. As I said I was unsure of how to handle this idea at the moment, so the seed sat dormant until a calling in the near future could give the needed nutrients.

I was transferred to a different HR position that I held as generalist for a start-up business within a large company. The tools and procedures I developed over the course of my time as an HR specialist now fell to me to apply in my new role as generalist. It was a great experience that I was on the opposite aspect of the equationtaking on the execution of the process , not the theoretical aspects of it.

While it was an amazing professional growth experience however, I was also experiencing personal development in the inner. It was because I had finally conceived after a series of natural and intervention-method attempts. Because I was in the initial stage of my IVF pregnancy I was unsure whether I was carrying two or three babies in the process of growing. I recall it being very stressful for my husband Nick and I but also very exciting as we began to expand our family beyond just the couple of us.

The uncertainty and hormones aside the fact that nothing was slowing down in the workplace. Being an entrepreneur inside a reputable company brought numerous unique challenges that exceeded the typical working day that would be for someone working in a well-oiled system. I had a difficult time trying to maintain my self-care of progesterone shots and frequent visits to the doctor as well as sleepless nights and the growing discomforts associated with creating new lives on the inside as I built an entirely new structure within my workplace. (I'm certain that you've been thinking this or similar thoughts in the past: "Will work ever be sufficient to allow me to concentrate on my personal day?")

After a very successful pregnancy and birth, we welcomed our first baby girl called Olivia. We were so happy to have achieved this milestone and also to see an active and healthy life. full party! Because my husband and me share the similar values, we believed it was essential to Olivia to have a family member at home that would be there to support her to the best of her abilities. Our husbands and me were both corporate warriors in the same corporate parent were both very proud in our careers and work pathways. Because my position at the time was more challenging than his at that time, it was decided that he took a break from his career and work part-time, and I would work full-time. Even today my husband will tell me that this break, which was to have the child was among the most memorable moments of his life.

After that and I was able to continue working through the night and throughout the days, dragging my breast pump around to work, where I would hold an image of Olivia when I was pumping as I believed I was doing all I could for my family and Olivia. It's possible that this will be familiar to any parents reading this The truth is that it was an enjoyable time, however this was the most exhausting moment in my life.

A typical day of my working week would see me getting up from one of those two-hour naps I'd have after nursing throughout the night while sleeping with my baby. The alarm would signal the end of the sleep-deprived of slugs. After that, I'd start the day with an extremely quick shower together with Olivia on the bouncer seat or the co-sleeper when Nick was away. I'd finish my preparation of lunch-packing the breast pump bag, my lunch box and things, and then say goodbye to my husband and little (or nanny, when it was a professional day for us both and leave to work for a 45-minute ride.

In the car I'd make calls or pump myself up with my most-loved tunes and then transition from mother to leader team member. From the moment I arrived working, I was involved with my colleagues as well as my boss, colleagues as well as my laptop almost continuously until the call of nature came in a way. I'm sure you're familiar with this routine! It was also important for me to ensure that I was keeping the nutrition and hydration and supply of milk up to par. I worked hard to keep my work-related productivity and engagement up at work. I would take breaks to pump and call home to check how Olivia was doing. I'd like to say that the process was smooth however Olivia was having other ideas.

My little girl was the one who no one could hold or feed without difficulty, other than me. Everyone believed I was too protective or even neurotic when I would declare, "No thank you, she'll cry her face off," when others wanted to hold her.

"Nonsense!" they'd say, "I'm the baby whisperer I want that child."

However, Olivia would cry and scream as if it were her job. It's true that it was. babies are so tuned to what they want that anything that isn't in line with it causes a clash. What a wonderful instrument is this? How unfortunate that our relationship to our needs can be cut off from us as we get older? We'll explore the subject a bit more further in this book.

When I called home, I'd want to know what the situation was like. Oft, Olivia would not take the milk bottle from her mom for the entire the time. It's easy to imagine the "fun" the experience was all those watching her, and especially for me as I arrived at the door. If it was a particularly difficult day, I'd like to get out of work a bit earlier to allow Olivia, Nick or the caregiver, me, and my boobs , some relief.

Sometimes, things didn't turn in this manner so I would not be able to pump as often. After a long, tiring day and long commute, I felt as full as a water tank in the game of the playoffs the moment I walked through the door . The baby was crying. "Hike!" was shouted. Instant football hand-off, work uniform ripped away and a scrambling, hungry kid, looking for a nipple heading toward to the line of goal. "Touchdown!" the crowd applauds. After all the excitement, there's an euphoria for the mini-athlete who is drunk and milk-fed and the entire team of coaches let out a sigh and relax.

The evening routine (and I'm talking about the time that ran from 6:30 p.m. until 10:00 p.m.) consisted of full of chores, meal preparation and consumption, bath time routines and routines for bedtime. However it's a bit nutty, aren't we? There's not going to be any sleeping at all the night. While I was still in contact with my emails, I'd be caught up on work to ensure that I didn't stumble into a storm later that day. And then the co-sleeping began. which was a mixture of nursing and REM-failed tries.

It's alarming again! Already? And off we go ....

Then, fast forward to IVF second pregnancy around 18 months after. I'm working full-time while breastfeeding a toddler and I'm beginning to think about the next stage of my career. I loved my growing family, however, I didn't feel a love for my job. Human resources' role (God thank you to everyone working in it) was more akin to an enforcer of rules for me rather than any other job. Now, if you are in the same position, you should hold your judgment for a second. I am sure there are many skilled HR catalysts on the market and each one sees and approaches this job differently. In my case, I found myself in a position in which I was not a fan of the structure. It was as if I was limiting myself and others because of my style and abilities. I was wishing for a job that offered greater freedom and flexibility as well as more potential and possibilities. This was not a wish in the least. I was entrapped by my situation. It wasn't that anyone was trying to trap me - - I simply did not know how to shift my perception to become different from the norm or to realize my potential to grow in the future.

Thank God for the knowledge and the courage to recognize that I was unable to determine my next step by myself. At first, I was feeling like I wasn't in a position to figure out the next chapter of my life. Not even the next step I needed to take. Then, I thought of the little seed that had remained dormant. I sought out a coach to help me to get a handle of my career path and also to know what it would be like to coach for other people. Through my own funds, I engaged Stephanie Yost, my first life coach, to begin the process of understanding my personal life as well as professionally.

As a result of this I was able to realize of my desire to become an expert coach, like the person who was helping me become clear and change. I enrolled for CTI. Coaches Training Institute (CTI) and, while working full-time, started studying the basics and completing the required courses to become a full-life coach. Instead of trying to assist the client improve one particular aspect of their lives, for example, their job performance, whole-life coaches assist their clients look at the larger picture, considering their lives holistically before making adjustments. This was the time during my coaching that I experienced an epiphany (or breakdown?) that completely transformed my.

To maintain the high speed and the high volume of work that I was working at, I frequently went to training for coaches on weekends, when I was far enough away from home that I required an accommodation. I also needed to bring my own childcare for my toddler who I was nursing as well as being extremely pregnant, and also building the second baby. As you, I tried to be a good mom and be efficient at it. I never missed a beat at work , and it was at the cost of sleeping, and even fun in my spare time. I desired to be a mom who was present and wife, a loyal employee, and a developing human being -- both professionally and personally. It was exhausting and overwhelmed by the task of meeting the needs of everyone.

In the course of one of my coach sessions during one of my coaching trainings, we engaged in an exercise called a Future Self visualization, in which I was shown my future 20 years from now. I saw an iconic yellow school bus leaving with me waving my children on the bus, and saying, "Bye, mom!" In the vision they had gone. While it was an "memory" of children in school in my mind the fact that they left the bus signified that I had not seen everything. It had been twenty years since I last saw them and I was now an empty nester. The tears poured down my eyelids, when I began to cry at the thought that it was over and it was as if this new life I was creating inside me was leaving the nest. I'd never even looked at his or her face and yet the empty feeling of grief and loss filled my heart instantly.

I was aware immediately that my life had to change. Working all day long and not having enough time to my family and me ... the cycle needed to stop right away.

In my mind, I realized that I was headed toward that direction for a period of time, but I also knew that someone needed to pay for the expenses and support my family. My husband and me agreed to change roles. He would work full-time while I would work part time , while focusing on my coaching career , and transitioning into mother-bear-mode. This was not an easy decision for me to make as the ego component which helped build a career as a breadwinner and corporate pioneer in a growing business felt disappointed. It's possible to be feeling the self-esteem that the ego gives about the achievements you've had at this point. However it was a decision I made. Or in my case, it felt like it was made for me at that point when I took a look 20 years in the future.

This change was the conclusion of something, and also the beginning of something much bigger. I completed my coaching training and went on to obtain the full certification of a coach at the same time that I was pregnant with our second child, a child named Raymond. In the time I was on time off with Ray I attempted to create a coaching role within the organization in which I could fulfill my passion and serve the company in a different role. However, it didn't go as planned as it was an idea way before its time and the business required a committed HR professional who was more passionate about the job than I did.

With a heavy , grateful heart, I handed in my notice to leave my job as a corporate employee. I sprinted towards a vision which I hadn't thoroughly vetted at the time. I didn't have a business plan, nor any Rolodex with clients. Sure I had my husband's support as well as benefits and pay -however it was my turn to provide the food and we relied on my income to support our family. (Perhaps you're also worried of risking benefit, the money as well as the capacity to pay for the mortgage, while being a major weight in this game called life.) It was terrifying to leap without no assurance from the parachute of the corporate. But I knew what I wantedto accomplish; it brought me back to a line from the film When Harry Met Sally: "I was aware. I knew how you're aware of a great Melon."

After just two weeks of leaving I was able to land my first client, and never returned. It has continued to grow and is expanding and growing since the year 2010 thanks to the power of word of mouth and referrals. In the course of one and a half years, in addition to an entire year of coach education I was able to work with my coach to understand what I had to accomplish and who I had to be to help me serve in this role. The pull of possibilities is too strong to choose in any alternative way.

Do I mean that you need to quit your job in order in order to be satisfied? Absolutely not, in fact, contrary. My path took me in this direction. I quit my job at a corporate company to pursue my passion for life to ensure that you don't have to quit your job in order to live your life.

Let me make it clear It's not an insomnia-driven, late-night infomercial which claims,

"You too can be the same way like I am without ever having worrying again!" My struggles and development aren't over. My ego is still in play , and I'm not living my ideal life that I imagine with flawless choices. I am doing the things I'm inviting you complete. I'm always in the presence of the assistance of a teacher or coach in my life because I really need and want someone who is able to hold an eye to my own life and help me escape from my own personal story. Keep in mind that you'll see outcomes and relief as well as the strength to go on with your goal even when the fairy tale does not go as planned. it should.

There are endless options you can choose to make in order to be more content.

Chapter 3: Evolution

As we've read my story, it involved an unintentional leap of faith that was outside my comfort zone at work. But, not all scenarios call for such a drastic change to regain your life.

Get to know one of my customers, a married mother of one as well as an executive VP in the corporate world, whom we'll refer to as Rachel. Rachel struggled to find time to exercise during the course of a full workweek. She felt uncomfortable if she woke early to run, or running after work, as each of these options would mean the loss of time with her family. Additionally it was the most dark time of the year and she wasn't feeling secure running in the vicinity of work during bookends during the workday. In putting off weekend warrior distance, she wasn't reaping benefit from the release of endorphins that she so desperately needed on a daily basis. The idea of running in the office was considered to be a sin. So, what do you think her boss would say? What do her teammates think? Rachel considered herself a lazy indifferent, either a leader or an athlete because the piece that she was missing was not there.

After a discussion with her coach the issue, she decided that she wanted to take a run during lunch breaks for about a mile or so in order to test what she felt like and what kind of consequences she needed to face upon returning. What terrible events took place? None. There was not a single negative consequence for her running during lunch breaks. Everyone who saw it took it in or was inspired by it since she served as an example for others to follow when making an effort to become more holistic and whole that made her an effective leader at work. Every situation will be unique and if you don't take an opportunity it's impossible to have a clue about what's in store.

Imagine a life where there's enough time to manage your life in a manner you're passionate about. You're in a job that's satisfying and rewarding. You have time for family, enjoyable times with yourself and the unattainable "me time" that we hear about on Oprah or Self magazines. You feel great regardless of whether it's the morning of Monday or the night of Friday It's all the same as you're finding a balance that feeds every part of your. You think this is a massive gag? I encourage you to think again.

I've worked with a variety of corporate athletes who are so committed to their work that they lose sight about themselves. I remind them often of the value they bring to the table by being committed workers and leaders. I also remind them that are doing their best work can with the tools they have and their state of mind. Yet, the call to be better. be better than is always available, waiting for the conscious willing, the able, and the capable.

It's like this: Often everybody else has the best of you. You're proud and happy to devote your talents and anyone else who requires you. Until you burn out. But what about the fact that you are still you? Don't you deserve it too?

Imagine this: You get to be the recipient of your own amazingness.

There's a place in which, when you're winning everybody gets a share. There's no deadline or job away. It's much closer than you believe. There are typically lots of questions and worries that raise their ugly heads whenever I talk about such things such as "work time harmony." I've seen everything, and perhaps some of these ideas that are often shared by my clients, resonate with you:

* "I cannot sleep well at night because I'm unable to turn off my brain from the endless list."

* "Because I'm so busy I am ashamed to take time to myself after work, when the family members are waiting."

* "I do not have the time to workout."

* "There aren't enough hours in the day to get everything accomplished."

* "I'm concerned that I'll regret never being present for my children"important milestones."

* "If I don't reply to every email, I become concerned that I'll not be able to catch something."
* "I'm an active person and my clients count on me"me time" isn't an alternative."
* "It is so selfish to have my nails done while I could be doing something with my nails at home."
* "If I refuse to tasks or people and tasks, I will not be seen as an active member of the team."
* "If I delegate, it will not be completed correctly or in time. It's more convenient for me to handle this myself."

If any are familiar to you, or you'd like to add your own personal hell-speak Be assured that you're not alone. You're a typical corporate worker in autopilot right now.

When you experience a moment like mine that wakes you up or you're in a state of slow progress, remember that it's normal to feel insecure about big changes. Perhaps you even believe that you're putting your needs first you're selfish. A lot of years of conditioning has made you believe that this is the case. I'd like to challenge you to see this as self-servingbut not selfish. It's likely that you've heard the phrase by the author Eleanor Brown, who said, "You cannot pour from an empty container." Unless you've got an amazing trick that I'm not aware of I'm certain this is the case for you too.

A myriad of emotions or concerns can arise when you are considering making modifications to your life currently. You have excellent work with good benefits and pay, and maybe a lot of things are going very good in your personal life. If that's the case what can you do to improve it? Why not let it become even more simple? Let's dream and explore what's in store for you?

This book will lead you on a trip. You'll confront whatever you're feeling and follow the steps necessary to live your ideal life that you enjoy in both work and your home. The strategies and steps in this book are derived from the methods I use in my work with clients on an ongoing basis in order to shift from anxiety and panic to tranquility and in confidence.

Chapter 4: Welcome To The World!

Before I accept an incoming client I ask them this inquiry about their life: "On a scale of 1-10 How much do you feel in pain?" One means the pain isn't too bad, whereas ten is the most severe pain you've ever felt. It's like being at the hospital of our lives when the doctor tells you to pick the emoji that best matches the severity of your pain. When I use the word pain, it's actually referring towards stress levels and also how you're handling it. If the person's answer is anything less than an 8, I'm not sure if we have to get together at this point. There is a possibility of spending a lengthy time in a state of trance and I've noticed that, except for the very painful, there's not much desire to change anything in your life. Of course, there are instances of exception, but the client's level of pain is the first sign to me of their consciousness about their situation.

If we are aware of the issue (the amount, the triggers, etc.) and we are aware of the triggers, we'll eventually be able to do something to alleviate it. In the absence of awareness of the hurt it's like a ghost placed the "kick me" sign on our backs and we are left to wonder what's wrong with us.

It is crucial to be aware of this. It lets you know the present situation to help you make better decisions to move forward. It's being alert about the present state of affairs to help shape the future states. What we won't do is to ask questions like the "why" questions from the past. Why am I following this pattern? What was the reason behind my decision? Etc. I'm not properly trained to help you see in the rearview mirror and analyze your life's past and explain why you're who you are. Counseling, therapy and other approaches are excellent alternatives to gather information and to even help you heal. Coaching can help you focus on the current state of your life and assist you in looking forward by guiding you through the road and make the right choice.

The next chapter we'll examine your awareness prior to taking action. "No pain is no gain," the saying goes however this chapter is all about "know the pain, and know the gain." You'll have to acquire that knowledge by expanding your awareness both mentally and physically before moving to take action. Also, we will look at the way you feel and what you're currently doing to address it. When you finish this chapter, you'll be aware of the triggers at work and your personal lifeand could be ready to take steps.

Acquiring Awareness

If you're in this book trying to find relief, then assessing your discomfort is a good way to begin. There's no need to take action based on this data; instead you need to know the current instant, knowing that tomorrow or the week before it might be different.

To increase awareness for you, just hold your hands over your heart then take a deep breathe through and out then ask yourself to the question below: "On a scale from 1-10 How much suffering am I experiencing?"

Log in and let a number be sent to you. Note it down. Then, take note of the areas where you feel the pain. It could be tightness on your jawline, a tenseness within your shoulders or or a little discomfort in your stomach. Maybe you're having trouble in this area and you feel headaches because you're thinking too much about the exercise. There isn't a solution that is right or wrong just consciousness of what's happening.

The reason that the body-mind connection is vital is that our body is our primary truth-seeking device. It is able to tell when something is not right long before we realize there's any "kick me" indication. I'm sure that you've discovered the evidence for this. Perhaps your immune system has a breakdown just in time to take that holiday you've had planned. Perhaps your skin is prone to an outbreak of rashes. Perhaps you're experiencing back pain, headache , or acid reflux is a problem for you due to your stomach strain. Every person will have their own version of the facts and yours could appear differently, based on the cause and the level of pain or the situation.

In the same way We have an amount and an physical clue to match the number. Let's suppose that for this exercise you're at a 10 out of 10. You're completely exhausted working life balance going out of balance and you cannot think of another week at this level of stress. You are able to check in with your body. Then, complete the phrase: "I feel this pain/stress in my _____."

The only thing you have to do now is to be aware of it. Accept it. Accept it. It's not necessary to stretch out the kink or try to get it out of the way. Simply notice it and note it down in case you wish to look for patterns in the future. The habit of noting the discord, and also the physical clue will allow you to overcome the reverse.

Let's look at the situation of Christi as an instance. Christi is in a conference, and yet again, the subject of the campaign is brought up. They're looking for a re-run. They've worked hard on this and the thought of more churn is an outcome of other people's poor decision-making. She's upset but she's not able to connect the dots to understand what she's feeling. She's maintaining her game face at the dozen or so colleagues at the table. However, her façade isn't really the whole truth. It's possible that she's staying cool during the conference however her body tells her that it's not so. Her jaw is clenched and she's white knuckling the pen in an effort to remain engaged in the discussion.

In the future, if Christi is conscious of her body's signals she will be able to work backwards in order to pinpoint what triggered the interaction and gain a better understanding of what she thought about it at the time. The body isn't lying. It's all part of the game of awareness.

Fighting Overwhelm

You are aware of this tenth place you're in right moment, and you can feel the ache in your body. It's possible that you've even referred to it as "overwhelm." I'm sure I've experienced overwhelm, the feeling that "there's simply too much to be done, and not enough time and in the end, I'm not likely to be able to meet the expectations of other people or myself anytime very soon." Overwhelm manifests within your body in exactly the way the other triggers do. Perhaps it's a feeling of breathing is sluggish, as if it's an anxiety attack in miniature. Maybe you're sleeping less, because your brain doesn't shut down due to the list of things to do. Your body is telling your body your "truth" that you're not doing anything right however, over-abundance is a lie or a tricker.

Overwhelm can cause problems that don't exist yet, like its counterpart, Worry. My father has this quote from William Ralph Inge, "Worry is the payment of interest on the plight of others before it is due." Although it's very real in our lives, it isn't actually happening at this moment. It's typically a sign of the anticipation of what's coming in the near future (the big-ass list of things to do) or maybe it's the result of soaking in the wrong things in the past week (in the past). It's not happening at this moment in time.

What can we do to reduce the overwhelm? One of the most effective ways to repress it and anchor yourself to the present is to use conscious, intentional breathing. Our breathing is already on autopilot (thank God for that). However, to focus fully on our breathing is magical. Every second is a slow-down. It's not a novel approach at all. For instance, the practices of yoga meditation, mindfulness, and even sports involve breathing. If you're in a state of discomfort it is crucial to recognize the pain and be aware that the overwhelm is keeping you spinning all over the place, not the present, which is where you are supposed to be. Breath is the way to return to the present moment.

It is a technique known as breath awareness, where you do not attempt to manage your breathing at all instead, you simply be aware of its speed without judgement or an agenda. For me, I find myself slowing down and concentrate on my breathing when I practice breathing awareness. You can test and see if this is working for you.

One of my preferred methods of controlled breathing is square breathing, also known as the breath with four parts. Inhale for four seconds and remain for four minutes and exhale for four seconds, and then hold the breath for 4 seconds. Repeat. This can be done during an event or during a road rage incident in which you are tempted to shout or even lose it. Nobody needs to know the exact actions you take to keep your cool. Your breathing is enough! It's easy, it's instant and almost unnoticeable.

A method I use to keep my attention on breathing exercises in an office environment is to draw the square while I count to myself. One side took me just four minutes to sketch. The second, third and fourth sides each take just four minutes. Then, I draw around the square and continue to breathe for a few seconds. It's very relaxing and helps me focus on the present moment since I must focus on the drawing, the counting as well as the breathing. There's no room for stress in this moment. There's it's not a time to fret about whether I defrosted the meat before dinner, or that my list of things to do is growing due to the fact that I'm taking part in too many meetings.

This time of peace although fleeting at times can be so beneficial to understand what triggers cause you to be in a state of mind. When you feel like life is taking you by the hand (and you're not driving the life) A little bit of mental sanity can assist you in seeing the road ahead clearly.

Be aware of your values

I've talked about triggers a few times. They're any event that can knock us off the track. Everyone has issues but I'd lie if declared that my goal in life is not to be set off. Sometimes I'd like to be entirely Zen however, how do I know what is important to me if not triggered at times? We're looking through the through these triggers to discover what is important to us at the core values. When we were in coach training at CTI we spent a lot of time thinking about the person we are at the core of who we are. We do not decide our values. They aren't morals or values but rather they are inherent to us.

Let's look at a scenario working. There is a member of your team who always shows up late. You've come to accept the same from them however, you're still irritated when they arrive with a litany of excuses 10 minutes after the hour. What of your values are being challenged? Punctuality? Respect? Productivity? It could refer to any of a variety of different values. The need you feel isn't being fulfilled and you're experiencing reactions. Then comes the paintake note of how intense it is and how it is manifesting within your body. If you're in need you can breath through it and focus of the importance that was taken away.

It is important to note that you did not act differently even though you've been breathing with more focus. It's still just aware of what's happening. We'll go over values more in depth during Chapter 6, and the best ways you can use them as a sort of compass. We just need to be wide aware of these values, even if we do nothing different.

Take a moment to take a look at what if the pain level was at five. I've said before that this number could be a sign that you're not yet ready to think differently. You are currently in the mode of tolerance. Even tolerating provides us with information and lets us know what we value. It is important to consider what you're tolerating, and then ask an inquiry regarding trade-offs. For instance, if you're tolerating a coworker who is always late every time you get together, but you're not really being triggered to 10 points, then which alternative do you prefer? Perhaps you want to keep peace, so you prefer not to address the tardiness. If you are prone to continue with old habits it is possible that you haven't examined your habits and determined what's most important to you.

How does this information connect to managing time and work balance? It is impossible to change what you're ignorant of. It's not something you would do at work, would you? Start looking issues without a solid base of the knowledge you have? The pain scale can help us determine the best course of action. It allows us to determine whether an issue merits fixing immediately, or if we're willing to put up with it for the sake of something else more important for us right now.

The awareness I have discussed until now tends to be reactive. Let's recap. You're in pain and are paying attention to the place in your body the pain is manifesting. The pain was caused by something, and you're looking for the potential value it could be fighting against. The next tool you'll employ will be an evaluation (or an inventory) of your existence, to ensure that you are completely aware of you and the level of pain you are experiencing.

It is the Wheel of Life

I always include an image of the "Wheel of Life" in my new client's packet. It is a great way to gauge how fulfilled you are "Wheel of Life" is a way of taking a picture in time that shows how satisfied we are in various crucial areas. You might have seen variations of this wheel in the past but it might be an entirely new concept. Even if you're an experienced user of this method It is always a good idea to check where you stand now and make a fresh start, as fulfillment is often changing.

I've modified the old model of this wheel using my experiences with clients as well as the categories that we work with the most often. My most recent version includes twelve categories:

* professional
* Money
* Health
* Romance/significant other
* recreation and fun
* Family
* Friends
* Support system
* personal development
Physical environment
* self care
"Higher Power"/Higher Self

To make the wheel, create a circle, then cut it into 12 slices as if you would cut a pizza pie. Each slice should be labeled on the outside of the wheel by each of the category listed above until every slice is labeled. For a downloadable worksheet of the Live Full Coaching version of the Wheel of Life, please see the resource section of my website: (http://www.livefullcoaching.com/book-buyers/).

If you look at these categories, you're trying to figure out your position in each on a scale of 0-10 which is 0 as the lowest and 10 being the top. Be aware that this isn't a game of quantity it's a qualitative game. It's the relation to the particular category that's important. Let's take a examine the subject of money. There are many people who, according to societal norms, are at the upper range of income and yet are frightened about their finances and believe they're never enough. They rate them as low in the group. There are a lot of people who are within their budgets and are in a good financial relationship.

They might earn less than their fearful counterparts but they still rank this category extremely. It's not a test you must pass , but it's an aspect of awareness that allows you to look at the complete image of your highly active life.

If you are about to complete the assessment Try not to think too much about the process. Simply fill in the numbers very quickly, depending on the first response you have to each of the categories. In the beginning there may be a hint of tension or guilt showing up. Do not allow the "shoulds" come to the forefront. Refrain from being a slave to the idea that "I need to do more," or, "I need to cut back on my expenses" Make an effort to eliminate all the other similar could-a, should-a and would-a thoughts which aren't actually helpful. Put them away and take a look at what your satisfaction gauge actually tells you.

Also, remember that even if you give something as a 10 does not mean that you have any other goals in this particular category. I have many perfectionists in my coaching, whom remind me as well as their clients to never rate anything 10 out of 10 because there's always the possibility of improvement. They'll affirm, "I'll give it a 9.5." Yes I understand this. But you're not depriving yourself of anything when it's a true 10! If you're truly happy in your chosen field, you should consider giving it the 10. I guarantee that it won't remain there long as the moment your perspective shifts as does your evaluation.

Here's a short the summary of each one means and the purpose behind the rating system:

Career. It is possible that you have a job you love and which is satisfying, even though you are working seventy hours per week. If it's the job you've always wanted to do and you're truly satisfied, then you should evaluate it with an extremely high score. On the other hand, you might be a powerhouse with a title however, your job does not speak to you personally. In this case, evaluate it according to your needs.

Money. It's a fact that, despite what you think we live in the world of an absolute necessity. What you think about how is done with money (earning it and saving it and spending it, giving to charity, loaning it and so on.) each one of these influences the way you feel about it. In a scale of 1-10 what level of satisfaction do you feel by your relationship to money? One of my most favorite things to complete is asking the question "If you were your money's lover what are you doing to treat the person you love?" Are you trusting your money? Or do you check your bank account each hour to check whether the money "came home" already? Have you got a number of rules that create anxiety? Consider money as an individual How do you imagine money would react to your mood? Consider this section in terms of satisfaction in that relationship, and not in terms quantity.

Health. It is true that this can always be improved and you could face specific personal issues or goals. But, you should look at the present and determine what your satisfaction is with regard with your overall health. A different example would be a bodybuilder who has the body's fat percentage of 3 percent, who is still extremely upset about their inherited high cholesterol issues. Compare that with a 70-year-old who doesn't win any competitions but is content to live a full life, running around independently and is cancer-free. Yahtzee!

Romance/Significant Other. You could be happily married or divorced. You might be single and feeling alone. Or, you could be single and love it. There's no one-size-fits-all scenario in this case; simply take a look at how happy you feel within this group. Also, I have to share the time (and only once) I received "What does it mean if you are in a relationship that is distinct from a significant other relationships?" So, you could rate the two separately, but no judgement in this case.

Fun and recreation. It's true! It's the fun you've said you'd like to make more time for later Let's look at where you are at today. It's possible that the annual renting an island splurge isn't enough. You'll feel more satisfied with every day laughter at this point to help ease the burnout. What ever it is it is, we're not yet figuring out a solution we're just evaluating.

Family. Like the category of friends below is all about the how well the relationship is run rather than quantities. Think about your immediate and extended family connections and those who are most important to your life. Are you satisfied with these connections?

Friends. Consider this in like you thought of in the prior category. When I first evaluated the category I gave it low due to my focus on the lack of acquaintances I have. But then I realized I love and cherish my few friends like family. Then I realized that this wasn't a "quantity" game! Your score must be determined by the satisfaction you experience from the friendships that you've built.

Support system. I have added this category because I realized how crucial it is to give as often as you give. Who are your advocates and your system of support in your hectic life? This could include physical support such as cleaning the house or childcare, as well as emotional and mental support like the life coach, group leader or therapy. From a perspective of leadership how do you support yourself at work? Assess how satisfied you are with the support system you currently have.

Personal development. It is crucial to examine this area by looking at it from a different angle that isn't directly related to your professional development. What are you doing to develop your skills, interests, or interests? What challenges your body, mind, and soul, beyond your work-related training? Assess the satisfaction you are currently experiencing by completing this section.

Physical surroundings. This is the most difficult of areas. Consider where you spend your most time, whether that's an open office space or a house that requires repair and a car that you like (or cannot stand) with a long drive either way. The amount of satisfaction you feel from where you're physically is dependent on how your surroundings affect your energy and mood. I'll give you a short personal experience.

When I quit my job as a manager I was a mother of a newborn and a two-year-old who was at the house with a nanny, while I set up an enterprise of my own. I had one nursery on just to the left side of my office, and the opposite bedroom to my left and I couldn't coach via phone as my children would listen to me and experience temper tantrums. I would leave and coaching in my car to create a space to make a difference in how my customers' lives. I thought about renting space above the local Starbucks. My physical environment score was low! Yes, I was in an excellent, safe house, but the effect that it had upon my work was such that I was compelled to relocate. We quickly found a house with an office that was detached, and I'm currently in a high-scoring 10/10 in my physical environment. I hope this article will help you evaluate your physical environment score in assessing your personal circumstances.

Self care. Yes, it is a separate category. I've added it to the wheel in order to maintain that it is in the forefront and to increase its significance, regardless of how you determine "self take care of" (or "me time." You might find that there's some overlap however this is the case to any of the categories. Self-care could mean massages or mediation, CrossFit, or hiding in the bathroom with a People magazine for 10 minutes. You can rate how satisfied you are in this particular category according to what you believe self-care to be about you.

Higher Power/Higher Self. This is a category that relates to how you define what is higher than you. It doesn't matter if you consider God, Christ, Source, Buddha, Mother Nature The Universe, the universe, general energy, the Law of Attraction or your most authentic, highest self, it's something that is greater than you taking a breath and spouting it in this world. What's your relationship to this group? Let's say that you don't have any belief at all and you're completely content with that. If that's the situation, you might wish to place it higher because you're solid in your beliefs, even if they aren't the most popular ones.

After you've completed each section, mark the document and take a look around. What are the strengths? What are the potential opportunities? Keep in mind the principles we've discussed:

* Quality and relation is more important than quantity.

* Don't think too much about it.

A ten does not mean you're no longer pursuing goals.

* Look out for the--, could--, and would-haves (an indicator the inner voice of your critic might have been the one to rate this time).

We're still in a state of awareness People! But there isn't any action needed. If you want to, turn the piece of paper you scored each category into an origami bird, and then fly it through the window. I'd like you to be looking for new themes, surprising and confirmation. What was it like when you completed the questionnaire? Sometimes, people are down, possibly due to an unfortunate event in their lives or maybe because they've just cut off the blindfold, revealing their perspective on the world. Some of my corporate clients' initial reaction is to think that their career is only one slice of pie due to the fact that they spend a lot of time at work, or thinking about it. There it is you, my dear readers you are a reality you're a dynamic multi-faceted person with plenty to give and get beyond work.

Each of these categories could affect one another. Each can affect the other like an ocean that lifts every boat. If you have given "money" an excellent score, for instance maybe you could spend money on other areas where you're not as satisfied like "fun" and "support system." However an unsatisfying score could hurt others for example, the time the inflatable pool's float suffers tears when six children are able to jump onto it. It's important to recognize the areas that are performing well, as it is important to be aware of what is holding you back. There is a lot of good that can be accomplished when you use your strengths to your advantage. Take note of your own perception of this moment in time , and then try to be gentle with yourself.

For a quick recap the past few weeks, we've accomplished quite a bit in the first step. It takes confidence to be honest, sincerity, and a willingness to even notice an "kick me" sign or even start to get rid of it. It's been taught how awareness affects your physical and mental health and how breathing can help us to be present and give us a sense of the present moment. The things that matter to you, like your values, bring you to tears. You've noticed how dynamic your life can be. These elements look like looking through the fun-house mirror with facets of your life to gather data for you to make progress. Once you've mastered that you're suffering, you're able to identify the benefits. In the next chapter we'll look at what's next for you, with the awareness machine.

Chapter 5: A Way To Effective Choices

You've learned how to stroll, awake, through your world. Now that you know the direction you're headed, you are able to make better decisions isn't it? But not right now. If we were to jump into all sorts of activities currently, it might result in some shifts however you'll first have to slow down to speed up.

I can see that this may be counterintuitive to your "get the job accomplished" personality. In fact, I've observed the majority of clients feel intimidated by their own opinion of what they see on the Wheel of Life -- to the point that they're dragged into an Nike commercial and immediately begin taking action. Moving so quickly may get results. In reality, you'll achieve results. If you'd like lasting results that are in complete agreement with what you truly is, you should think about a few things before taking actions.

This chapter you'll take that knowledge from earlier and move towards acceptance. Imagine accepting as ownership. You may feel something that resembles an emotion, but you cannot be aware of it and take it as your own. When we acknowledge what is the case, we can choose our attitude prior to taking a step externally. When your internal game is in sync it will reflect in your actions or the outer game.

My clients have heard me say, "powerful choice," often. The word does not always refer to a extravagant move, however it can indicate that you are completely committed to the decision you make. It's a sign that you control the item 100. You're fully assuring it, to speak, rather than just half-assing it. It could be an example of getting to work on time however an internal customer made visit and asks to know if you're free. In normal circumstances, you'd reply, "Sure, I have one minute, so sit down." But we all know that it's never only a few minutes. Even though you're trying to help and be available in times of need, you're aware about the way you feel when you are able to give away all those minutes.

Then, you make a wise decision and tell me, "You matter, and the same goes for this subject. And you are worthy of my complete attention. What can we do to schedule an interview to a time that will satisfy both of our requirements?" Sounds impossible, you think? But it's totally feasible, so let's look at the steps to take to accomplish this with confidence and dignity.

Attending Acceptance

This chapter is about the inside. Making a powerful choice is an inner job. With your awareness as well as "body experiences" as evidence, we are now able to examine the effects of our decisions. There's another step to be taken before we can act out of awareness and this is to accept. Acceptance does not mean that we've settled or we're stuck. It's just a sign that we're engaging in a process of taking full and complete ownership of what's happening now. You've probably heard the abbreviated quote from Carl Jung, "What we do not like, we will continue to." What we don't want to confront tends to expand or become louder. If we're not aware of something that is true, it's bound to be a pain in the back until we face the truth.

There's a little cleaning to be done in this area -- some internal cleaning to ensure that we don't lay the new carpet of strong choice of dust and dirt bunnies. Keep in mind that as your coach I'm not here in order to repair the past you've had or to fix your present It's not that sort of cleaning up. Your coach will view you as naturally inventive as well as resourceful and complete (that's the CTI cornerstone) This means you're not damaged, and are not in need of being repaired. Everyone is springboarding from a solid foundation. But, the inner energy or funk that might be circling around us must be taken into consideration. We are at a point where decisions are made so let's make sure that space can be as clean as is possible. With great energy comes the best option.

Let's look at one of the triggers for frequent flyers we have previously discussed. It is possible to tell that you're addicted to nicotine. You're reminded of it whenever you have a desire for a smokey snack and there's no way to deny it. If you don't acknowledge your addiction, you will not be able to take the next step with a vow to stop, so go purchase the pill, and then follow the effects.

Another instance: during the day, you're aware that you're double-booked. It's evident since your calendar is a gruelling reminder of the layers of appointments that will never be attended to by you with all your attention. If you're stuck in the "what's-it-all-about-is-it" mode aren't going to be carving out empty space any time in the near future.

What do we do from now? Start with something you feel motivated and eager to tackle rather than something that is based on a sense of obligation. Perhaps the harmful habit of smoking is too overwhelming and difficult to face. Let's not choose that first. Find a low-hanging fruit which you'll feel satisfied having accomplished maybe that's clearing your schedule. Whatever issue you decide to tackle this will give you the motivation to tackle it and complete it. Before we take action we should do some internal game-playing with our self-esteem.

I have a tendency to judge myself harshly often. I coach and teach about this, but since I'm human I fall into the trap of ego. I may be depressed or feel depressed about not having achieved goals, an injury that keeps me from achieving my goals in CrossFit or yelling at my children due to my standards being too high. This isn't good to me. And when the knee-jerk response or the off-feeling starts to creep in I feel like I'm a failure.

In these instances I'm the one who is the most affected by an uncontrollable emotion or self-deprecating behaviour which isn't helpful to anyone. My self-esteem was a hindrance. I felt righteous or right and, darn it that someone else is going to be paying! However, often (almost all the time) it's me who is the one to pay for it. One of my coaches Dana Williams, to look at areas that need to be forgiven. The act of forgiveness helps us accept whatever is happening. It helps bring peace to the place that you may have missed in your quest to act. If I am in a moment where I'm not in control (snapping at my children) I remind myself to take a deep breath, keep an eye on my triggers and what's going on and to let myself be forgiven for my human-like moment.

The forgiveness of a wrong doesn't make it right Just as saying that you're sorry that you were late to a scheduled meeting does not make you appear on time. But, it does open the way for acceptance and a different choice for the next time. It's a decision to heal instead of a choice to make a right choice (again thanks Dana!). The more we work on awareness and acceptance and acceptance, the more likely will be able to block the anger outbursts and adapt before they happen (#goals).

Every single thing that happens on the Wheel of Life, whether you give it a score of zero or a 10, originates from the an inner game. Inner game is a phrase used by many athletes in their practice before the gymnastics event or the crucial swing at the hole 18. For them, and for us, it's a way to are able to achieve our goals based on where we are focusing and not on what we would like to achieve.

I'll go into more detail about this concept in the future and to clarify it for you, I'm asking you to look at the true meaning of the following expressions that you're in a bad state of mind because you "got in the wrong place at night" and a chance encounter was a disaster because you "got off in the wrong direction." This perspective that we practice is the lens that we view the world and assess the situation around us. The mindset we adopt or our mental narrative affects the actions that occur. We are in control of what happens next , so it is crucial to begin with our attitude. It is the choice we make about our inner game that affects our external game.

After all this acceptance and awareness What can we do to change our perspective? Grace is the key to gratitude.

Being grateful for all that is happening for us is option to turn your life from being a mess to amazing. Here's a real-life story to share about the importance of the attitude of money and.

The coach I had been working with was my coach, Jeanna Gabellini, on my business style, personality, model, and obviously money. At that time, I was caught in the middle of a financial slide. The terms of corporate payment were shifting towards ninety-days, however, my bills were still paid weekly. I noticed that my savings were dwindling in an effort to cover the expenses of our household and I began to get anxious. I'm the person in our relationship who is steeped in abundance and has a faith-based mentality, so when I'm stressed that we all worry. When my financial well was dripping the water well in our home dried up. No joke! The water was all dry and I couldn't help from engaging in the laugh-cry-laugh cycle as I raised my fists in clenched hands at the absurdity of the Universe.

Did you remember the question earlier regarding money at the wheel? I asked "If you were a lover of money and you were to treat him or her, how would you treat the person you love?" Let me tell you that in the scenario which I had to be in, cash is at a distance from you! I was pressing refresh on my internet bank account, and chasing unpaid invoices, and all with the feeling of constantly texting my spouse, who could be cheating, "Are you there yet? Are you there? What time are you due to return back home? !"

Jeanna suggested that I keep a gratitude keep a journal of everything that I do, with the exception of money, to shift the vibe of F-you that my financial situation has created. For the next 30 days I would spend every day creating a gratitude diary my gratitude for the small and major aspects of my existence. A few examples follow:

* "I'm very happy with my wood-burning fireplace and the rest of the cords of wood that are stacked around my house. It helps

keep my home and my family warm, and it makes me smile."

* "Thank for the new Tahoe the big and secure vehicle that can transport my three daughters securely and takes me to my clients during the winter."

* "I'm very grateful for my fitness and health. I'm able to rise each day, workout, and feel great. I am grateful for the well-being of my husband, parents and kids. We're all healthy and alive."

As I type these words I am filled with satisfaction. My breath is deeper, more enjoyable and more relaxed. There is a slight tingle on my face as well as a warm feeling in my soul. In the past, this method helped me live my life. Not from my physical demise however, it saved me from the mental state that was draining my financial well-being, my happiness and, presumably my true well.

Do you know that , after the 30 days of gratitude journaling, money started flowing in like a flood water hydrant during a hot sunny day of the city? One of the benefits of gratitude is that it is acknowledging what's already happening in the world. It's already there! Therefore, there is no need or desire or feeling of awe when we're thankful. This is pure appreciation that will ease any resistance to accepting. When I could truly recognize the things I already had money came flowing easily.

It required me to wait for 30 days to complete this case, but there's no ideal formula to explain this. Continue to practice gratitude practice and observe what changes occur for you. Do not set an agenda. It's not easy however, being attached to the result as a measure of success can cause more opposition.

There's a different approach as focusing on what you control, for instance your thoughts. The difference is what you intend to do in comparison to. your expectations. The intention you have is your own internal. What do you want to feel? What's your strategy for emotional stability to deal with what's in store? It is entirely within your power to direct and direct. The most common mistake is trying to influence the result. Expectation is an external thing. If you think that if I do this, I'll anticipate this. This is a trap that can cause many disappointments. Here are some examples starting in the office.

Workplace Examples:

Goal: "I'll host an associate celebration to demonstrate to my team that I care about them. It'll be a great feeling for me to keep going on this idea regardless of what they think of it."

Expectations: "I'll host an associate appreciation event to make sure that my staff will be content and appreciative of me for it. Their response will be an honor to me, and it'll aid in retention and engagement."

Personal Example:

The intention: "I'll invite my friends to join me for a dinner since it's good for me to be open and inclusive. I'm a huge fan of giving and give my time and energy together."

Expectations: "I'll invite my friends to a party since they'll feel so thankful and we'll have a blast together. And then they'll invite me to the future gathering."

Note how the action of the mind is not a part of external reactions? The expectation is 100 % dependent on an external reaction that you can't influence. I'm sharing this information with you in the hope that you can find peace and tranquility by focusing on what you are in control of and getting rid of things that you aren't able to control. It's the Serenity Prayer really nails it: "God, grant me the courage to accept the things that I cannot change, the strength to make changes to the things I canchange, and the understanding to recognize the distinction." I typically begin my day with this prayer with my kids before they board the bus. This helps them recognize the difference between intention and expectations.

The majority of people dislikes the kind of exercise I recommend because they think I'm demanding total control. Be happy for control freaks! Me too. Develop your inner-game mindmastery, an intention

Ninja! That's the new game. You can observe that we haven't done any different. We're being different.

Your Inner Critic

As we remain within our inner game circle I'd like to shine the spotlight into the darkness for a brief moment. It's not easy to remain optimistic all the time and be able to rely on the knowledge that we have the ability to influence our thoughts. It's not the goal to never experience any dark thoughts or moments however, rather to) become aware) accept our awareness and finally,) take control of this new perspective.

I compare it to the thoughts that float into your mind when you meditate. You attempt to be Zen, breathe and close your eyes and then you're done! The list of things to do appears as a movie reel from the past in your head. The sound of the projector's click and the static sound track remind you not to complete all the things you've set out to complete. You're not always in control of the thoughts that come to you but you can control and redirect them to ensure that they don't hang out for too long.

Let's try this with your own inner critic who wants to be there and disrupt your day. I was taught this technique through CTI However, there are many methods available to help you control your critic.

Imagine that you are in a meeting and you've been handed the responsibility of a new project. You're overwhelmed by the tasks that's on your plate. The voice in your head is a snarl with the same message: "You aren't good enough to manage this." It's awful! And you believe that voice too. Your face is squinting up, and a sour feeling is felt in your stomach. What can us do when you hear not-so-supportive voices?

There are some steps to follow. In the beginning, you must record the phrase or phrases that this particular voice often uses to express its opinions. For example: "You aren't good enough." Then, you would like to characterize the voice by giving its mannerisms, clothes or posture so that you can imagine this as you listen to its recurring chant. Name it! It could be thought of as an older version of yourself or your parent, or even a real person in your life. But you'd like to name it to give it its own distinct identity. Change it, so that you can get an accurate sense of the presence of this creature when it is in your vicinity.

There is a positive aspect that is hidden in this darkness. Your inner critic may be trying to help the cause, or help you to avoid something. Lovely, right? But, in the beginning of a visit, it may not appear so charming. This is the perfect moment to take a look and discover what's good about this. There are many reasons to believe that the critic is simply trying to get you to try to be more efficient, be sure that you're not wasting time or avoiding tasks you can finish at a high quality, etc. It might bring back memories of a nice but dysfunctional aunt who was at Thanksgiving meal, however it's crucial to be aware of the fundamental message.

Next step to keep your inner critic to be engaging in something else that isn't. Give your saboteur a favorite hobby. When you're not in your jeans, what do they do for pleasure? After its wisdom-filled words are deciphered and brought back to its goodness and positive qualities, you congratulate the inner judge and let it go off to perform the task it is most excited about without your permission. It'll leave happily because whatever the other thing appeals to it. You then return to your life with a more positive heart and a more focused. Don't allow the inner critic to distract your progress.

As time passes, you could encounter several voices. Do this exercise for each one -They have their own approaches to get their way and a variety of lessons to learn from them.

When I first began the practice, I soon started to realize my loudest inner critic. It would be triggered when I was seated to read a book in which I was not planning to gain knowledge and was instead absorbed in entertainment. The voice would ask, "Why are you relaxing? It is possible to do many other productive things in your spare time, such as running five miles."

As I heard this voice I was able to only see was a large-haired image of me from the 1980s wearing the Wonder Woman costume: hands on her hips and a cape that was flowing in her back (even even though I couldn't sense a breeze) With a sharp face and a voice. I called her Overactive Superhero. She was unable to be bothered by the thought of me not achieving anything every single day. A novel to read to have amusement? Guffaw! She'd prefer me to exercise my work ethic and improving myself by other means. Roger that, overactive superhero! Thank you. Now, you can go to work and do as many pull-ups as you can! Then she went off without a step on her red-booted steps.

Consider where you might be hearing this voice in different areas of your life for example, within your group as well as your neighborhood, family, or your circle of friends. We would like to change your relationship with your inner critic by recognizing it of acceptance and the power of decision-making. For a refresher of the actions you need to consider for yourself:

* I can be able to recognize the voice once I can hear the voice.

* I will take the lessons learned, learnings or a the message of protection.

* I'll send the inner critic to you with thanks.

* I will make a conscious choice about the way I play from this point onward completely embracing the decision.

The aim is to reduce the influence this voice exerts over your life over time, and not to block it from ever showing up. It may be heard at least four or fortytimes per day. Then it will lose its spark. It's the same as it's a move to a tune you've heard before. You're working on it, feeling some gratitude, and getting the power back. All inner-game magic!

(For a downloadable worksheet please visit my website:

http://www.livefullcoaching.com/book-buyers/).

The next section, we will utilize our inner compass to investigate deeper by identifying the most important things to us in terms of our values.

Chapter 6: Defined The Values You Value

We now know the way that our internal dialogue is translated into external actions. Let's be more specific about the underlying causes of these triggers and feelings to be better equipped to deal with the raging waves of our lives. In this regard I'm intentionally not analyzing any of your previous. However, you should be aware of the signs that something is off and what you can do to correct or honour these issues. In this section, we'll explore the mindsets that stand impeding our ability to live in total honesty and openly and discover how to make use of our beliefs and values as a guide for a powerful choices.

As we have discussed in the previous chapter our values form the heart of who we are. An authentically fulfilled state is one where we make decisions that coincide with our values, which are the items that are the most important to us. It is possible to judge other people for their beliefs if they differ to your own. It is possible that you have to give your power to, or withdraw without a reason frompeople who do not adhere to what you value most. It could be in the form of blaming on them for the reasons you're unhappy or making them responsible for the actions that cause you to lose your day. Truthfully, the source of your happiness isn't at the hands of others. It's up to you build it and keep it! Each of these ideas is beneficial in relation to the knowledge we've acquired since, when you're fully awake and conscious it is easier to decide how to apply your belief system.

Clients often ask for the list of values they want to include; This way, they are able to determine what is essential to them. This can be useful in a restaurant where you glance at the menu and begin to swoon over the choices that are presented in writing. It's better to explore your values more naturally. The most powerful, open-ended questions can be a fantastic method of revealing some feelings and triggers as well being able to identify the values that underlie them.

Here are a few questions I've asked prospective customers to assist them understand certain values that could be at the root of the responses.

Tell us about your most cherished pet pet peeve?

In what situations do you think you're the most critical?

Do you remember the moment you last got angry or frustrated at someone.

It's possible that these questions are on the controversial aspect, however I like them due to the fact that triggers are usually closer to the surface, and there's no need to dig for these triggers. There is a wealth of knowledge in the dissonance which can aid us discover our own values.

If you've been battling anxiety and stress due to overloaded nights and days it's easy to search at what's wrong. Actually, you aren't looking at all. You are abusing these moments as if you were biting, nastier horse flies on a hot summer day. Instead of grumbling about these instances, let's take a look at what they're saying to you. It's like the public service announcements from your critic.

Perhaps the most irritating thing you have in the workplace is employees tell you, "Yes, sure, I'll take it" with a sense of excitement and determination But the results show up months later, following the deadline was missed. What does this is a source of concern about what matters to you? Maybe you value commitment, punctuality following through, commitment and honesty. Perhaps it's something different? I like to write each thought out in a stream-of-consciousness exercise to see all the threads. The words may be different to different people. only you know what the words you write mean. The thought process on paper can help you see things clearly.

Here are some questions about the other side -Not things that bother you, but those that make you happy -- that can help you to capture the essence of your heart. This is what you call resonance.

* What was your most proud moment in your life last year? From your life to date?

* If you were free from limits to your talents or time or money What would your most secret (or not-so-secret) goal be?

* If you had an alternative career to this one What would you choose to do?

• Who are people in your lives you admire? What qualities of them are you looking to imitate?

The same process applies to looking into your narrative and identifying qualities that come to the surface. Was your most memorable moment from the past year revolve around the work you did, for instance, the team's project was completed in a blaze of glory? Maybe the fundamental values involved include teamwork, completeness and appreciation. If the moment you were most proud of in one of the most important moments in your own life happened to be the first time you had be crystal clear about the value you is ascribed to. Was it love, family or the legacy?

I'll share with you an experience from my own life that gives an illustration of how the term or value could refer to different things in different contexts to various people. When I attended an instructor training course for coaches shortly following the birth of my second child I was in a discussion about the most important moments of our lives to establish our beliefs. I chose the time of the birth of my daughter as a moment that was new to me. I was expecting my second child and about to begin the second cycle. A colleague of mine mentioned that the birth of their own child was their best experience also, and as a result, we agreed that "family" is the most important significance that the birth stories of our children.

When my friend spoke on her birth experience, she said that family for her was "the more the better," and that it very unique to have her entire family members in the room for the delivery. I think she mentioned that the birthing party was around the double digits. I was imagining

I'd be to feel heart-beats at the thought the same kind of experience with family, in the way she defined it, was not satisfying to me. After having gone through IVF that involved a lot of pushing, prodding, and little privacy, the thought of the peanut gallery accepting our baby was not acceptable. Family to me was affection and intimacy. Family was a very special thing for us both even though the specifics of what we were looking for in it varied.

While you search for answers to these questions using instances from your work as well as your personal life, look for common themes. You might notice that love appears everywhere, or that other themes, like family and honesty, integrity and so on. are constantly surfacing. This is how you know that you're ringing the tuning tones of your values. Do not worry if you can't make a tidy elegant list after having journaled for about ten minutes. The most effective way to organize your personal values is to allow your checklist to expand organically as time passes.

Although the questions can be provocative questions to think about, your life's troubles and fears will offer more details right now. In these instances, you can go back to the lessons of Chapter Four which helped you observe your feelings. You can apply this knowledge a little deeper and use it to label the value of a thing.

If we're triggered by the rudeness of a person blocking us at the intersection (you're listening to one of the members of the road rage club right here) Instead of acknowledging that we're angry with rage, burning on the cheek and probably screaming, search for and acknowledge the value you feel was infringed on within you. If road rage strikes me typically, it's the value of consideration or respect I feel like I'm being knocked down. Evidently, I'm judging other driver, without knowing the entire background. Perhaps they're experiencing an emergency in their family, or they've heard terrible news and require to a place quickly.

Let's admit it ... during the midst in the present, we're not attuned to their demands, nor are we disconnected from our actions. I'm sure there's more to come on how to deal with the judgement monster. In the meantime, you can make use of the trigger as a way to determine the underlying value. The same respect value that was lost in the crash will be celebrated in a different positive, more positive situation. We will be able to recognize it when it surfaced, too.

To illustrate this procedure Let's say that we currently have a list of three to five items with the knowledge that the list will expand as time passes. You can classify the values in order of importance. However, this isn't required, as the importance could change with time or in accordance with the circumstances. What happens when two values compete against each other? Ah, the timeless work-life balance routine. You are really concerned about following through and making sure that you complete tasks for your team in a timely manner. Also, you are very concerned about being a great parent and going to your child's Cub Scout awards ceremony tonight. These values chains -- following through commitment, accountability, love family and follow-through -- all are important to you. How do you decide?

This is why I'm a huge believer in making a short-term decision, and then putting your to the test of your priorities at any moment to determine which of them has priority. What is the most important thing for you at the moment? What would grab the attention of this instance - or the Scouting activity or outcomes? Be sure to trust your heart and your brilliant brain and it will work regardless of. If you make a choice that is strong and make the right choices, you no longer are dependent on the situation and you're most definitely not in autopilot. If life is taking over you it isn't your responsibility. Let your perfectionist enemy! You need to slow down in order to speed up. If the conflict between opposing values leaves you feeling frustrated and raw, take a look at what's important to you today, in the near term.

In this instance of Scouts against. deliveryables Scouts could prevail because of the importance of the ceremony. When it's a typical meeting of the den Perhaps you'd be able to send proxy members to help. The deliverables will be completed, but possibly later in the night and the following day. It's time to revisit your contract with your family members, your self as well as your internal clients regarding expectations, one step at an moment.

I like making short-term choices that respect values since you can choose which value you want to honor at the moment, instead of. needing to think for years on a single value. I also enjoy changing my opinions. This is the reason I'm not a tattoo-wearer (this isn't a judging of tattoos in any wayI'm just a person who knows myself). If I'm being honest with myself regarding the moments that appear to be whimsical I'm not going to re-create the plan. It's possible that you disagree, and that's fine for me, however I'm offering this option to give your tired mind a rest from constantly being a slave to ideas that might not benefit you.

Outside of consciousness and naming values on their own You can view them as integral to your personal GPS or compass of sort. When I discovered that my two most important values are flexibility and freedom in relation to flexibility and freedom I view every choice through this lens. I feel more content when I'm embracing these values, rather than when a structures are in the first place. Keep in mind that I love to be able to make changes in my mind which is why a job or pastime, or job that requires a strict rigid routines isn't my thing. I was once a commodity trader and the daily routine that brokers called, opening markets trading, closing the market and books and so on. was like a imprisonment for me. For many, this is their ideal dream come true. I say to each to. Concentrate on what is most important to you, and take note of the choices you're making which are in line with your values.

There are instances where freedom isn't the winning factor in my game plan. The circumstances that cause this aren't common however I'm thinking about the instances in which I made the difficult choice to challenge it. When I make the choice that option, I give myself complete control, which feels more like a choice and more like a choice.

This is one of the myth-busting ideas I'd like you to try out regarding the balance between work and life. To achieve it, you must have an inner game awareness and focus shift. If you are able to approach the balance knowing that you cannot achieve everything You have to trade something in for another thing -- it's how you're going to feel about your life. If, for instance, you feel that you have to skip dessert since you didn't go running the day before to burn off the calories Consider whether the decision is a necessity or is an acceptable trade-off. Wear your best pants and choose. Tell you, "I'm choosing this -the dessert or this job, or this person --

because I'm honoring a certain value." Know the value. Zero people here. Bravo! Sometimes, you'll feel an intense reaction to the decision. You're aware that it's not right, yet you make it nevertheless. What did you think of that? My request that you slow the pace down and reduce your expectations of others until you are able to take the pulse of your own values. It's true that you'll have to pay today or in the future, and my goal for you to make certain that you're winning because the positive ripple effects of your success will be a dividend.

What happens if neither option does you feel good about? What happens if quitting work earlier feels awful and not attending Scouts is equally awful? Decide what you want to place on the moment, knowing well that there will be different decisions to make before sunset, and opportunities to make various decisions. This is an invitation for action to no longer be an opportunist and become the one who wins your beliefs every moment of the moment. Are you prone to making mistakes? Don't worry about it. Choose to do it differently the next time.

It could be that I'm telling youto "Suck it up buttercup." However I'm asking you to believe in this procedure. If you're unable to be sure, start acting differently and gather the evidence for yourself.

It could be a bit uncomfortable away from what you're familiar with -- running the maze of life on autopilot. Take care of yourself during this time. If you're judging obstacles and accidents and accidents, you're less likely to be able to look at the situation. Take a look at the lessons learned with an eye of curiosity since curiosity and judgement are not compatible. Do it! Consider whether you're truly interested, or are looking for proof to prove the notion in your mind that you have already believed. You'll always find what want to find.

I often tell the people I work with about having "one that you are." Do not wear masks to work and then tear off the mask on your return trip in lieu of a different mask. Who are you as a person? This authentic version of you is the one who adheres to their beliefs unapologetically. Don't try to impress your fellow sheep. You must be yourself first, by recognizing what draws you in. Do more of the same thing.

Distress vs. Eustress

Sometimes clients opt to participate in coaching simply because their boss has told them they need to make changes. Feedback is a blessingIt's your choice to accept the opportunity and your decision what you make of it. 360 surveys, which are employed in many workplaces together with other surveys, are extremely effective in helping reveal blind spots and obscure strengths. Like all surveys there are advantages and disadvantages to these surveys. I'm trying to emphasize that, at the end of the entire process of executive coaching, I would like clients become more real and to increase their value system further.

Do you remember hearing you'd be more successful when you weren't all that much of you? It's true that I've been told this.

I'm too noisy, too optimistic and extroverted. whatever. The feedback I received used to be a sting. Now, by coaching that is based on self-love, awareness and acceptance I'm able to choose my priorities in accordance with my values and it's awe-inspiring. I'd like to share this with you! I would like you to get out of hiding. I would like you to cease being a people-pleaser, or a saver and instead focus that focus on your own authentic. The world is going to win when you are successful! You can't win if you're a confused actor trying to figure out which role you are supposed to fill when. Be yourself -- every one of you.

The salmon swims up streams to survive. I get it. If you have a value that is based on fighting, then embracing the values you hold dear becomes your guide to navigate through the water of your life more enjoyable way. It is possible that you need to be challenged and you're aware that the most satisfying experiences are difficult. As a three-time natural birth veteran, I am completely in agreement.

I'm referring to the distinction between distress and eustress.

Returning to the story of salmon. I'm confident that if I were the ESPN announcer of the legendary salmon run of Alaska and could converse with any of the salmon along their way up to spawn, they'd be frightened because their existence is dependent on it. If we're not looking to only survive, but are looking to be successful then we can do it by overcoming challenges in moments as well. Eustress is the positive stress you experience prior to a thrilling task. It's that feeling you experience when you are at the start of a race or when you are about to step onto the stage for a speech at your sales event. Your heart is still pounding from your chest, and your breath is sluggish as well as racing. The excitement of it all and the accomplishment of the target is well worth the excitement.

If you'd like a more in-depth worksheet on how to clarify values and make decisions accordingly, see the reference page in the back of this book, or visit my website:

(http://www.livefullcoaching.com/book-buyers/). We'll learn more tools that will help us flourish even more as we move forward. In the next section, we will place you in control which will allow you to be more than ever to live your life to the fullest.

Chapter 7: You Are The Boss Of You

It's time to turn up the volume of powerful choices that will make you the most important person who will benefit from these decisions. For the real-world actors that are around this chapter will be an opportunity to make a difference. It's time to get your power back, both in regards to both your actions and the perspective. This chapter will help you'll learn and implement methods to alter your inner game, help you improve your game's actions on the outside and establish rules and boundaries to help you take care of yourself.

Perhaps you've measured your accomplishments based on the achievements or accomplishments you've made until now. Perhaps you've measured it in terms of the qualities your boss or colleagues at work have noticed about your character. I'm asking you to redefine what success is by embracing energy as the new standard. What is this referring to? It means that your own performance (before, after and during actions) is the new measurement of your success. What are you feeling when you make decisions, setting your goal or creating your list? What do you feel like during the course of the project, or when you're doing something? What do you feel like after the project is completed? While there are shades gray in these answers but there's a fundamental that you should ask yourself to determine if your on the right path Do the things you're doing drain or fuel you?

Your self-care and levels of energy are the most important aspects you should be focusing on now. Have you ever tried driving in a car without fuel? Even the gas-free Tesla requires a sleek recharge station. What's your equivalent to charging and fueling? Even before our gauges are screaming "empty," what are doing every day and out that deprives us of energy? The time is now to tell "no" to ever more of those activities or do them in a creative way with a fresh viewpoint. Stephen Covey, author of 7 Habits of Highly Effective People has urged readers to develop their habit of "sharpening your saw." It's impossible to continue doing things like sawing if we do not make time to recharge or sharpen our tools. We're all aware of these tips in our heads, but we've not trained enough to create the muscle memory that we require. If we did, we wouldn't have been discussing burnout.

Let's make the first step to decline. Another option is to simply cut off the work and let it go off your to-do list completely through delegating, negotiating or any of a variety of alternatives that will stop the drain on your energy. There is a chance that you'll be able to disagree. It could be that you believe that if your "voluntold" to perform a task in your job, or when a circumstance at hand requires you to take specific measures then you're not in a position that you can choose. In addition, your belief system about saying no can numb your mind, and prevent your from taking an decision other than grudgingly moving forward.

There are other approaches to the problem.

Let's consider an example of the house first. Personally I'm not a pro in the area of organizing and cleaning. It takes the energy from me, and I'm more inclined to stay clear of it as much as I can in order to conserve my energy for the things that I like, such as budgeting (yes that's the truth!). Therefore, for me, I assign these tasks to service suppliers as well as "barter" time in exchange for services. If you have the option of hiring someone to help then do it. If you are struggling with money you can exchange favors with your friend or family member who is a pro at this sort of thing. Whatever excuse you could think of I'm sure there's an answer that is suitable.

For entertainment, let's pretend that there's no solution. You're stuck with the same version of grunting. There are methods to make it more enjoyable or even enjoyable. When I'm performing a gruelling chore like cleaning or organizing I will put on my headphones and blast out my music like no one's business. It's the music that I can plug into my eardrums , which makes me feel calm and amps into high gear to the "woo-hoos!"

So, I decide to make cleaning more enjoyable or at the very least, more enjoyable. I'm less exhausted in this manner even though the job is considered to be a essential for me right now. While the "what" happens but it's that "how" I decide to complete the task that keeps me going.

From a business viewpoint, we're too often presented with goals, projects or lists that aren't our own and that we are compelled to follow them. My hope for you is that you have the power to decide your own "what" as well as the "how" every step of the procedure. Do you think you're able to refuse to work for the boss? Remember, you're the boss of your own.

Let's try this. For example, suppose your boss has asked you to reduce the number of employees you have while keeping the current workload on your team.

A few people might be enthralled by these acts however, let's pretend you're unhappy with these actions. As you place the dipstick into your tank of oil the situation is looking down and dark. You might think that there is no other choice than to go ahead with your plan. However, you're probably underestimating the power of your brain. When I say brainpower, I'm referring to your intellect along with your ability to make choices about your thoughts, which transform into actions. As negative as your thinking and your perspective are, the more negative your tasks and experiences. Luckily for us all that the reverse is true also. More positive you're thinking and your perspective is, the more optimistic your work and experiences.

Then you can break it down. What are the key elements of this project that make you feel exhausted? Perhaps, for instance, you are struggling to let others know that you have left the team (or even worse, are no longer employed). Maybe you're having a difficult to disappoint others, and you'd rather work 14 hours a day instead of saying"no" to some one. Maybe the idea of not being able to deliver to your employer is painful as you value your contribution and efficiency. Maybe all of the previously mentioned (or some other scenario that is not named) takes away your enthusiasm. Be aware of the details and dig deeper to find out why they hurt. There's gold!

Think about, "What can I chunk down and delegate or refuse to?" Using the example above to determine headcount, what can you do to collaborate in conjunction with Human Resources or others to make changes to your players known? Are there any other people who are really skilled at this? Can they guide you, coach you or even tag team with you? Do you have a different approach to deal with the situation?

If you are able to maintain the current workload and operating your business in the normal way, consider ways to be able to say, "No, not yet and not today." There could be others with strengths in this field who could take on specific projects or tasks (inside or outside of your team). What are the best ways to re-evaluate your terms so that you feel good about it? Take a look at the triangle that includes time as well as money and resources (e.g. humans capital). If one side of the triangle shifts in any way, the other sides will be affected. For instance, if the timeline is cut, how can you can increase the investment in cash or of human capital to allow that to happen quickly? As an administrator, you have to think about and make choices and the resulting consequences.

Keep in mind that it does not matter what I included or left out as scenarios that could be considered. The most important thing is to think about some tough open-ended questions that do not require an answer that is either yes or no and then you examine each possible option. While you evaluate each option make it appear as if that's the option you've chosen to pursue and then evaluate your level of energy. Did it improve? What can make it even better, simpler to handle, more energetic?

I'm sure you don't want to be a disappointment to anyone. However, If you're tired and performing poorly due to it, the chances of being disappointed by others are much higher in general. If you are adamant that work is taking a toll on your life at home Does it matter what you're "winning" in the workplace when you're unhappy every day? Consider the situation this way: you're not being honest with yourself and you're the number one customer. If you're satisfied then everything will come together much more easily faster and in a manner that will leave you with more energy.

After you've analyzed all options Let's say you have to complete the task There are there are no "no's" permitted. I know, I'm aware. I've already walked you through each of these choices. But, I'd like to show you what's feasible even if you believe or think that you're not in a position to make a decision.

It is the next thing to contemplate the kind of shifts in perspective that you can create. When you're experiencing dread or exhaustion and dread, that's the way you'll feel about all actions. However, if you take on an entirely new perspective for a few minutes, such as testing a car before you purchase it, you'll discover that there's an entirely new experience to be enjoyed during the same commute to work. Here are some questions you can explore for a fresh viewpoint:

* What is the best gift to me or others from this particular experience?

* How is this going to be more simple than I imagined?

Where is the excitement, the joy here?

* How could this experience become my best teacher?

There is no limit to this method, but it is important to search for a fresh perspective and look at it from a different angle. Consider, for instance, the scenario in which team members leave to cut down on the number of people in the team.

What's the reward? Perhaps it's an opportunity solve the issue of talent or give people the chance to pursue a new interest by moving somewhere else.

How could this be more simple than I imagined? How about tapping into people who could help to guide you in this. You could assign the job to someone else. It might be more beneficial the experience on the sidelines instead of taking on a leadership role since it's a temporary issue.

Where's the excitement, the enthusiasm there? Perhaps the enjoyment level isn't as high However, what could provide more energy is to recognize them and express gratitude to them for their services. It's possible that finding the right way to express your gratitude, the words and the timing that you feel most comfortable with will help you to gain more energy.

What could be the best teacher I could ever have? There's no reason to anticipate these events however there is always something new to learn from the process. For instance, there are new perspectives on the transparency of empathy, openness or skilled communication.

You can always find an answer to serve you , if you believe it's accurate. So long as you're believing of this being "it" as well as that "it" is a snare the hell out of you, it is bound to. Therefore, you can either change the way you react or shift your perception. In either case, you will gain more of the things you concentrate on. Why not select a more positive either action or thought?

Self-care is self-serving or self-centered?

There is a chance that you are in the category of those I work with who think, "taking care of me is selfish." Maybe you work extremely long hours, have to travel to a distance that is astronomical or work in a global job that is never a day off. If that's the situation, I'm sure that the idea of having to take time off from work or family obligations is just selfish in your head. Perhaps you have been taught over time that it's been instilled into you to prioritize others over your own needs (after all this is the way that "good" soldier do). Perhaps you are suffering from guilt as a parent or spouse if you are involved in me time during the time between the semi-annual vacations (when you're likely to be connected or online at all times).

Truth Smack! I'm glad to shout out from my hills that neglecting you is selfish. What is the reason I'm speaking such foolishness? because you are not able to provide anything worth mentioning over time to your work, your personal life or the planet when you're miserable and stressed, sick and drained or even burned out. It's easy to believe that your friends and your family members are doing the best they can ... But how much time? What's next?

This is your new motto"Taking care of me" isn't selfish. It's self-serving. Remember that the moment you're successful, everyone benefits. It's true for boys as well as girls! Get ready to get your tickets for Self-Service Show. Self-Service Show.

I myself went through 12 year of Catholic school, and putting myself first was a lot of reprogramming. I also need to be reminded. I don't mean to offend my faith-based education, but it wasn't particularly popular to indulge in "self" in any way.

Add that to my desire to please, be generous and give back at work and throughout my entire life and you have the recipe for burning out.

I often look to nature to find the perfect model of self-care and cycles. It is necessary to let the winter dormancy pass winter to allow the world to blossom in spring , and flourish during the summer. In the evening, flowers stop their blossoms, and creatures that sleep during the day are able to replenish themselves. It's normal, it's natural and necessary. When our egos, brains and external influences interfere it is a sign that we are not following the rules.

It is important to recharge at the workplace as well. Our sleep-deprived global roles require naps every day. You decide when and the best way to take these breaks However, some examples could include:

* Actually, take an "lunch hour" to eat , or take a walk. (Geez!)

* Do not log on until your kids have gone to bed. (Gasp!)

* Have something "fun" on evenings on the weekends. (Guffaw!)
* Do not work on weekends, provided you're not in call. (Gulp!)

I don't care about whether you practice all of these or a combination between them or even create your own self-care routines. Simply start doing things that feel good to you , and quit doing things that do not.

I know that the sun never rests, however it's a massive burning star that's bound to go out of existence at the end of time. On contrary are a part of the earth and require replenishment and rest just like all living things on the planet. Cycles, baby. It's all about the cycles.

But, there's no negative news. Sometimes, our passion and values are recognized in a way as we confront issues that eventually take us away. We talked about values in depth in the previous chapter. If you're allowing the rest of your life to dictate how you spend your day at the cost of your energy that you're doing an act of disservice to yourself and, in turn all those who is around you.

I'd like you to assess your current beliefs regarding self-care by putting your beliefs according to a rating scale from 1 to 10, with 1 being"nothing at all," 10, being "hell sure":

It's a shame whenever I do my own thing.

* I'm not able to look after myself.

"I don't have enough funds to care for myself.

* I don't have a system of support (e.g. the significant other or work culture, childcare etc.) that allows me to take good care of myself.

Find some common patterns in your answers. What are your biggest issues? What do you have your greatest strengths? If you look back over what you have learned from the Wheel of Life, you may find strengths that you can use. For instance, for the majority of executives I work with there is no financial issue. Thus, they are able to invest a little money in solutions like hiring a trainer to help with the workout they need or hiring an infantsitter so that they can go on a mini-vacation.

If workplace culture is your issue, I'll reiterate that you are in charge of your work. What you do to create this moment or shift in perception is yours to decide. While you wait for other events to shift that you are unable to make your own decision. You can claim it! In our current day and age particularly for the generation of millennials working life balance is becoming more popular. Of of course there are deadlines and team meetings, and many other obligations. I'm not suggesting you not pay attention to all of it. I'm just saying that where there's a desire there's a means.

Healthy Boundaries

I would like to discuss limits with you. Perhaps you are feeling the discomfort of your current limitations or boundaries that you face in life. It is likely that you're embracing some strategies to address the. In this article the concept of boundaries is a good all-time best friend. They form the basis for the self-care that we are building.

They form an element of our pool's walls to allow us to be free to swim in our newly-defined, self-care water. They act as the safety nets to keep us away from the cliffs, from where there is no way back. We can apply "no" through the use of structures that allow us to remain in the self-service lane on the road of our lives.

I counsel my business clients identify which areas of their energy are greatest and lowest throughout the daytime. They can then write those times down in their calendars online to be used as "sacred times." Are you not someone who is a morning person? Don't schedule meetings until 9:15 a.m. Don't feel like you're burning out at 4.30 p.m.? Make sure you are not meeting after 3:00 p.m. And, now I can totally know what to do when events pop up and people ask you to every conceivable thing. Make sure you check your energy levels. Consider, "Is this draining or unnecessary?" Then, say "no" or delegate. Do you think this is a game-changing task? You can make a smidgen of exception and declare "yes," invoking the decisive choice that you'll draw inspiration from sacred times and bring a new outlook to it.

If you're allowing to allow the everyday "river dance" throughout your sacred hours, you're allowing everyone to dictate your schedule. There is only one person accountable in this situation, and it's you. If you're totally fine with it, that's acceptable because you're not exhausted. Be honest with yourself and understand your boundaries and your intolerances.

T-Tool

Sometimes, we're trapped emotionally. The happy words written in the mirror's lipstick will not magically alter any thing. This tool I'm going to discuss has been crucial for my own changes and also the shifts for my clients. It was invented in the work of Rebecca Hanson and is called the T-Tool. I've employed the tool with clients over the years following my visit to Rebecca's Law of Attraction training center.

1. Select a subject on which you're feeling stuck and want to be able to change your perspective.

2. Draw a huge Capital T onto a letter-sized sheet of paper.

3. On at the very top create the title of your topic.

4. Write "I don't want/do not like feeling" on the left-hand side of the top of the T

5. Below, make a bulleted list of the emotions associated with the subject that you do not want to experience. Continue until you are able to not think of another.

6. On the right-hand side on the right, note "I would like to feel."

7. For each of the bullets to the left write a list on the right what you would like for your body to be feeling instead.

8. Create a big "X" across the Don't Want side , and Fold the piece in half, so you only be able to see the Do Wants.

9. Make the three affirmations below for each bullet point:

O "I am currently working on ..."

O "Higher God/Universe/God ... are currently in the process of ..."

"I enjoy it when it happens." ..."

Here's an illustration. Let's say that you're stuck with a view about your boss. You are feeling a bit over-managed and unappreciated. Work is difficult and you believe, "If I just didn't have to report to him, my life could be much more enjoyable." But the truth is that you can't influence this reporting relationship immediately unless you decide to quit your position. You can't control what he is doing, however you are able to determine your actions. If you're not yet ready or willing to go, or you are uncertain, you need to modify your behavior and regain your power.

The first topic could be "relationship with the boss." To the right, you will find "Don't Want" feelings may be characterized as being micro-managed, not appreciated, not valued, frustrated, stuck, etc. After these have been reframed the reframe column to the left could read as empowered and appreciated, admired and peaceful or. After you have written all the Reframes then draw an "X" across the left-hand list and do the three sentences every time you write a new bullet. You will notice the difference in just one minute! As you continue to do it and practice, the more you'll see the changes becoming swift simple, effortless, and long-lasting.

The only instance I have observed that this isn't working is when a customer really isn't ready to change. In this instance they're still tied to their beliefs and don't have the motivation to change their perspective. Remember the question that was asked earlier Do you want to be perfect or do you need to get better? If you're ready, take a test run and then let the shift take place.

We've concentrated on the game inside, and the best actions on the outside will be based on the new, grounded and well-adjusted position. If we were to begin setting goals and make decisions without first working on this first it would be only some movement. Now we're prepared to attempt an exercise to set goals using our new perspective and new approach to make goals be realized.

Corporate warriors or not, you've likely encountered or used a version of SMART goals (specific goals that are measurable, achievable realistic, time-bound and realistic). It is possible to visit the resource page to learn more about the background of its development. At CTI I discovered that there's a more engaging version that is backwards known as TRAMS that allows you to be more involved in goal setting.

T (thrilling) What's exciting about pursuing this goal at all? What are the steps involved in taking it on and what does the it look like when completed? Finding the excitement is crucial. The standard method to "just take it on" may feel dull and boring.

R (resonance) R (resonance): That's where your values are in! What values will you be able to honor in pursuing this objective? Following the extensive research we've done on values you'll see how crucial it is to link the dots and understand what objective is in line with who you are.

A (accountability) A (Accountability): Who is will be your cheerleader in pursuing this goal? This isn't the whip-cracker that yells at you when times become difficult, but someone who lifts you up regardless of whatever.

M (metrics) M (metrics): This is where you'll define the success criteria that you normally write down in a typical goal-setting exercise. What do you know what you've accomplished successfully? We've already learned that the addition of a metric to measure energy level can help to dial the process even higher.

S (specifics) What is the best way to ensure we achieve this objective? What is the particular strategy and steps it requires? This will help you define the strategy to take forward.

Check this method against the usual corporate goal-setting , and take note of the differences. It is possible to doubt whether this kind of optimistic goal-setting approach like TRAMS could be useful to the workplace. However, I have seen it firsthand and know that it is effective: I tried this approach while I was HR manager of a new company. It helped individuals shift their thinking and focus on their heart and mind connection to a goal far more than the typical SMART exercises. Let's take a look at a practical example of a requirement to reduce the budget of 30. Most budget cuts is emotionally charged for people in certain ways. In this scenario, let's assume you're not a person who supports this goal and you are having a difficult finding the motivation to participate with energy. Even if the objective was implemented with solid business logic, you could be able to feel resistance. Here's an example TRAMS in this scenario.

T (thrill) Although it may not be exciting in the moment, I enjoy the excitement of engaging with people who are skilled at this and can encourage me to explore my thinking outside of my current thinking. It's also exciting to be able to complete a task by using creative methods.

R (resonance) This is a way to honor my commitment to the team as well as the company by creating the budget that will meet all of the needs of everyone, including my personal. I'm also honoring freedom as I'm able to refuse to do things that don't have a mission or don't provide the greatest return on investment for the company. I'll conduct myself in a manner that is respectful of my ethics and values of responsibility to present myself as a strong leader to serve the company.

A (accountability) Accountability - I'll inquire with Paul for his opinion, because he's been successful in the past and I have faith in him.

M (metrics) M (metrics) - The SWB (salary and wages, as well as benefits) and spending projections and project scope. are all in place by the time of the deadline (specific to this goal).

S (specifics) bi-weekly meeting with a traffic light scoring approach in relation to the above metrics, until the deadline , which is 90 days away.

It is likely that you have noticed changes as you are moving forward, and that the steps you're putting in place reflect an genuine, aligned version of you. Although it is powerful to be the boss of You We'll reduce the pressure in the coming chapters by expanding your support system by incorporating the most powerful partner: Your higher Power.

Chapter 8: Begin From Where You Are

It's like riding a rollercoaster with highs and lows as well as downs and ups as well as twists and turns. There will be a point in the journey when we get caught in the downward loop and stay in there for a bit too long. In the middle of the loop our life isn't pleasant and we are trapped in a state of being not at our most optimal. In the bottom loops, we are prone to anxiety, boredom, apathy and workaholism. This book will assist you to get through those lows swiftly and effortlessly. Whichever of these states you're currently in, you need to begin where you are in order to get to where you want to be.

Where are you now? What is your opinion on the moment with respect to what you would like to be? What is the best category to describe your current life situation? Are you bored, floundering through life, constantly busy or are you just constantly working? Are you not motivated and wasting your time not paying attention to your priorities, or simply having a difficult time balancing your life? If so, whatever you are in a bad spot this process of setting goals will aid you in turning things around.

From Boredom From Boredom Enthusiastic

The best advice for anyone who is constantly bored or is stuck in an unending cycle is to determine what you would like to achieve and be responsible for getting it. Boredom is a sense of being bored with whatever you're doing right now. It is triggered when you feel you have no options and you're stuck doing something you do not want to do or are in a position you do not want to be. Everyone has experienced periods of time where they are into a slump and loses the focus of what is important but the kind of boredom that I'm trying to tackle is a continuous lack of interest that can lead to the sensation of being trapped. This is a state that you feel as uninterested empty, unfulfilled, and lonely. The excitement seems to elude you and you do not feel the motivation you need since you are spending most of your time doing things that don't satisfy you. If you stay in this condition for all the time could result in severe health problems, such as depression. What is it that will be that you need to do to bring this about? Wouldn't it be nice to feel a sense of excitement when you reflect on your daily life?

The word "enthusiasm" is used to describe excitement, novelty and adventure. It is not common to use the word "enthusiasm" to how someone conducts their lives, however we'll defy the rule and go ahead and apply it. There is a profound satisfaction and positive energy that is reflected in the word"enthusiasm. It is a way that is filled with joy and happiness. Imagine for a moment what a happy life is like. This is the kind of feeling you will get by mastering the process of setting goals.

In order to break out of the rut and to live an active life determination and discipline are crucial for you to accept. It is important to determine the goals you'd like to achieve and who you would like to be in order to establish an excellent foundation. You must be disciplined to get yourself out of your comfort zone. It is possible to do this when you are aware that passion is on the other face of the action. In addition you must arrange a medical check-up to rule out nutritional or physical deficiency that could cause an unmotivated mood. If medical issues have been eliminated as a contributing reason for your moodiness The first step is to finish the exercises included in the book. The initial step that you must complete, that is the Planning Section, is where you'll reap the greatest benefits.

Between Drifting and Intentional

The expression "just follow the flow" is a perfect description of those in drifting. Drifting literally translates to being taken away by currents or water. The state of drifting refers to those who live with no purpose or direction. It's a condition in which you are "doing," not "being." The term "drifter" usually is a person who is engaged in important activities but lives in a state of confusion or not having a connection with their personal goals, or even their self-worth. Someone who is drifting might not be aware of it since the person typically has many activities, however these activities are usually planned by other people or to benefit others but aren't necessarily vital or important to the person. Afraid, but with no feeling of direction. The main difference between the Drifting Group and the Boredom Group is how much the tasks are satisfying to the person. Drifters don't necessarily feel dissatisfied with the work they're engaged in. They're not even bothered by them.

On the other hand of drifting is intentional. It's not just about doing, it's the determination of what is best and appropriate for you, and choosing carefully the things you do. It is based on your goals and dreams. It's a state that brings consciousness and concentration. If one lives their life intentionally they can make a decision about what they should do since they are aware of what they really would like to achieve. Intentional living means taking the passion within you to guide you throughout the day. If you notice that you are more to the drifting group, alignment and discovery are crucial elements in your plan of action for life. Instead of letting the forces of necessity determine your goals, creating goals that are aligned with your ideals is the best way to take the next step. Step 1 and 3 specifically, will illustrate exactly what you have to accomplish to alter this situation.

Between Busy and Productive

If you are into this category, you're probably a good person and have a spirit of giving, and a tendency to overdo things, and relaxing would probably be at the bottom of your list of things to do. In today's hectic world there are hands in many burning issues. Naturally, your skills and time are sought by many people, and you've got significant goals that can affect numerous other people. A lot of people in this state live in chaos and perform a myriad of jobs. They are able to take on every task that comes at them, however usually to the detriment of their well-being and health. The ideal is to transform your hustle into productive so that you can achieve balance in your life consistently. This means making a change to ensure that self-care is the first item on your priority list.

My opinion is that the most important factor that differentiates an unproductive person from a productive one is the ability to prioritize. Someone who has lots to do must ensure that he or she does the correct thing at the appropriate moment. They must choose to prioritize self-care first. Understanding the process of setting goals is sure to help. If you're in the latter category, then you might think you're too busy to complete the exercises, however there are steps specific found in chapter 3 which can help you with this aspect. The first step to learn about prioritizing is to set aside time to complete the book and all of the exercises.

From the Workaholic lifestyle to the balance of life

Everyone agrees that the hard work of a person is a vital element in achieving goals. The world applauds and praises people who are able to demonstrate a high level of integrity and with good reason. But when that working ethic is a cause for the neglect of self-care and other aspects of life, it becomes workaholism. Workaholism is a form of addiction that entails work and dominates one's life. To a lesser degree when you're in a way that work is more important than self-care, you're in danger of becoming an addict to work. Working-aholic tendencies are not the same as doing working hard. There is a fine distinction between them. The tendency to be a workaholic is a dangerous balance in life; while one can be able to work hard or even work long hours at times and still maintain a healthy balance, without causing harm to oneself or relationships. One thing we can be certain of however is that it can be difficult for those who have good morals to admit they've fallen into the trap of being a workaholic. Take a look at some most reliable dangerous, concealed, and ominous indications that you're an addict or have tendencies to work.

SUREFIRE SIGNS

I arrive at work early than the other employees.

I leave work much later than the majority of employees.

I usually work late hours.

My days are spent prepping for the week ahead.

I am not happy about having holidays because it could leave them in the back of the line.

I am willing to do the work that other people should be doing.

I wear my work load as a badge. Everyone is aware of my busy schedule.

I will not refuse work.

My schedule for work is jammed.

I work in the lunch hour and I eat lunch at odd times.

My family is worried that I work too hard.

Everyone tells me I work too much.

HIDDEN SIGNS

I long to work on days off.

I tend to prioritize work and try to avoid celebrations at the workplace and at home.

Work is often the subject of my conversations.

I work to provide an escape from my personal issues or the pain of grieving.

I invest more thought, effort, and effort in my work, but not as much as my relationships.

The only source of income and I am always concerned about losing my job.

It's hard for me to unwind when I'm not working.

I'm not one to hang with my friends, work is my preferred choice.

I am an absolute perfectionist.

I become impatient when need to wait for other people.

I'm not sure if others will support me or complete the job as well as I do.

I'm always running against the clock.

It's simpler for me to perform tasks than to teach others how to do them.

I am always busy and have my hands on many fires.

I am often multitasking and doing three or four things at once.

I'm very proficient in my job.

I am sure that the rest of my colleagues are busy,, so I am able to take on the additional duties.

DANGER SIGNS

I don't attend medical appointments when I am working.

My job is keeping me from getting enough sleep.

I am scattered.

I fall asleep thinking about my work.

When I wake up, I am thinking about my work.

I sit for long periods without breaks.

I'm feeling many stressors.

My family is not supportive of me.

My family is in need.

My family has been putting off asking me to attend events.

My family members are pleasantly surprised when I'm accessible.

My family is willing to make concessions for me or forces me to go to work.

If the bulk of these indications are true for you, then you should look at making the possibility of making some changes. Don't be content with the way you've been going. If you're not a typical workaholic however, you are aware of the need for some balance in your life, you should consider setting at least one goal centered around working-life balance. You should be able to visualize in your head of what a balanced life looks like for you, and you can apply that as your measurement of your success. This goal-setting process can help you do exactly that. It will show you how to be more holistic and beyond work and show you how to increase your efficiency in all areas of your life.

Balance in your life and living

At the top of the rollercoaster is the state of balance, where you're always doing your best. You're unaffected by the the trials of life and you are able to transcend the chaos that surrounds you. You are abounding and at peace. If you're at the point of balance in your life that is living energetically, purposefully and effectively, and are aligned with your desires and achieving your goals, then you're doing great and keep going! It's a state of happiness. When you are in this state, you are able to sustain your the success. Be grateful and continue to be a role model for others. I'm hoping that the knowledge contained in this book can be a supplement to the information you already have, and you discover gems of wisdom that will keep you on the right track of living your life to the fullest and helping others to achieve the same.

Maintaining The Success
To spark change isn't to give up; the momentum, you must change frequently.

If you don't find any other information from this book, take a note of this "Don't accept what isn't doing the job." If you're unhappy in any area that you are experiencing, make changes. If you do not address it, it won't change. If you continue to do what you're doing, you'll continue to get what you're getting. You must take a different path when you're not living the life you desire. You need to think about how you can make an improvement and then follow through according to your plan. This is the most basic method to achieve success. The plans don't have to be complicated however, they should contain the mental, spiritual, and emotional changes that are required to maintain the change. We don't want to just make a change, we are looking to be able to accept the change, master it and maintain it. Then you will be able to experience what I refer to as "easy life." Making goals that are effective is the best way to reach get there.

The definition of success is the achievement of an objective. However small the goal, you must achieve it and you'll have success. In this regard every person has success. It's an inherent element of our human existence. People struggle with their definition of success as well as the extent that they think they have achieved success. It is due to the fact that success is a private measure. It is essential to recognize that if you believe that you're successful, it's you who decides the bar and not others. It is possible that you have been influenced by the societal norms that define success based on popularity and wealth but it doesn't necessarily have to be the standard of success. Actually, the majority of people who succeed according to these standards believe this measure is merely superficial. They know the personal aspects of success and know how goals play in their success. I'd like to present this formula to you: whatever makes you feel happy Do it, and continue doing it, and it will result in long-term success. You will be able to determine what it means to be "happy," and you are able to define "success" within the same equation. Your job is to figure out what success will mean for your. The definitions of what is meant aren't static and will evolve as you grow older and change with the changing times. Also, you need to understand your own desires and your heart, and review that regularly. Stay in tune with everything you find. Do your best and achieve your best at what you can do in the moment.

The bottom line is that I hope that you feel happy. I want you to realize all your goals. I want you to build the habits of living intentionally and effectively in all areas of your life. It is my wish that you be content. There is only one life to live and it's too short to remain unsatisfied and without goals and dreams. The commitment to never be content, but to never forget the desires that are burning, to take on challenges with enthusiasm, be happy about the victories, and learn from your mistakes is the path to you. Let's get started now!

Step 1: Plan to discover What and What's The Reason

This goal-setting procedure is a method to modify and continually improve your lifestyle. Similar to other processes beginning this one is the planning phase. The planning phase requires the most thinking. It's about conducting the necessary research to determine exactly what you want to accomplish and the reason you'd like to get there. The time spent figuring out the big questions of life is worth it, since it's a crucial factor in reaching your goals. It's the investment you make in your own self-discovery, which creates the strategy and the energy and also lays the foundations for your decisions and creates a sense of ease in your life. The creation of vision statements for every aspect of life , by addressing these questions during the planning phase can save you hours of reworking and time wasted later. It establishes the framework and dramatically increases the chances of reaching your goals.

This is the first step of goal setting because it exposes the essence of who you really are (your talents) as well as what it is you would like to achieve (your desires). If you set goals that are rooted in your values and authentic self and your true self, you'll be more focused when you achieve your goals, and more joyful when you reach them. In this phase, you'll determine your goal/outcome as well as what success looks like, envision what you'll feel like after completing it, and consider the consequences of failing to achieve it. Create vision statement. It is important to define your beliefs in a way they can provide a solid foundation to set goals that are aligned with your core beliefs. In short, you're setting the course.

When setting goals, people often overlook the importance of the planning phase and usually do not bother to plan this step in order to go directly into execution. It's great to be enthusiastic about goals, but it's crucial to stick to the plan. We often are caught up in the rush to begin making our plans instead of making a plan for our goals. Planning can be either conscious or unconsciously either formal or informal either simple or intricate and quick or long-term. It's costly to skip or neglect this step. If you don't take this step, you're likely to be apathetic and whirl in circles and rework a lot of things or stumble later when trying to determine what you're doing. I guarantee you that the further in the process that your planning is completed the more likely it is that you'll either give up on your objectives or abandon goals that force you to stay in the same old routine. The lack of planning is the main reason people fail to achieve their goals. It's very easy to drift off course in the absence of a the direction and have a plan. If you discover it difficult to stay with the goal or simply not making progress take a look back at the stage of planning to review the WHAT and Why.

I'd like to warn that you stick to the WHY and WHAT, and not try to figure out how. A lot of people abandon their plans because they cannot determine all the complexities of getting them to be realized. This isn't the moment to make that decision. Concentrating on the HOW early in the process can lead to the eradication of desires due to fear. Avoid fear by staying clear of the how.

There are many exercises (Exercise 1-7) during this phase which are transformative. They put the spotlight entirely on YOU. Even if you do not complete the entire process of setting goals like I'd like to see you do be able to, take time to plan the exercises. The purpose in planning is come up with the vision statement (Exercise 8) that define your goals that you'll ultimately set. It is a time-consuming process when you've never really thought about what you want to achieve. However it's the most beneficial investment for your self, your happiness as well as your productivity. It will prepare you for prosperity for the rest the rest of your existence. In essence, setting goals like this will keep you motivated for the long haul when they are in line with your hopes and dreams. You must do this analysis to ensure that your messages are coming from you and not from what people expect from you.

Exercise #1

Review your current situation. This exercise will evaluate what's going well in your life, and what's not working. Make a notepad and name your document "Current inventory." Then, divide the sheet in two and on the left, title the paper "What's Working" and on the right side, name"What's Not Working. "What's Not." Think of the goals you would like to pursue and then place them on the right side. As a contrast, think about the things you're settling for in your daily life. What are the habits you would like to change? Make sure to place them to an appropriate side. After you have completed this exercise, don't be entangled in the realities of your current situation. It is a forward-looking approach to our thinking process. Your present state is actually your past. We will analyze this data to get an idea of what you're like and what you'd like to be. We'll utilize it as a benchmark to measure how far we've come.

Exercise #2

Who are you, or who would you like to be? Create an outline that includes "I are ..." in relation to your character" and the list of "I am ..." dependent on who you want to be. A second one should include the adjectives you admire in others , but you don't believe you can do or at the very least, confidently. Take a look at both lists and test yourself to see the similarities or what's keeping you from becoming the person you would like to be. Additionally take note of the way you feel about certain words, and which ones you're hesitant about including on your list. The list of aspirations is crucial because they can be transformed into vision statements and goals that can be used to form habits. Spend a few minutes to consider the following questions and then write down your results:

Which are the strengths you have?

What are your favourites and what are your dislikes?

What behaviors and traits do you want to change?

What are you most proud of?

What do you believe?

Exercise #3

The most common dreams are those that arise in the early years of childhood, or are frequent themes that pop up repeatedly. Begin to think about your desires. What makes you smile just by thinking about it? When you were a kid What did you think you'd be and be able to do? Even in adulthood What have you always wanted to pursue but stayed away from due to insecurity or ignorance? If you've experienced trauma that could have affected your vision, they will most likely be brought up during the exercise. Do not dwell on negative feelings and take note of your dream nonetheless. Now, it is time to remain positive. Write down the that you believe will bring you joy regardless of how absurd they might seem. A lot of times, your hopes might not look the way you had imagined them but they will be realized.

Exercise #4

Brainstorming session. You can brainstorm ideas about things you're passionate about. What are you truly looking for? What are you hoping to feel? What would you like to do? What is the best way to use your time? If money wasn't an issue then what would you want to have, to do doing, to accomplish or achieve? It's your chance to ponder, to drift into the realm of fantasy. Below are some additional questions to think about and record the answers to aid in the process of planning your goals.

Which new skills do wish to acquire?

Where do you wish to go?

What habit would you like to change?

What kind of car do you want to drive?

Where would you like to be?

Do you wish to find someone to share your life with?

What is the problem you would like to resolve?

What type of business would you like to begin?

What are you looking to accomplish?

What are the changes you would like to see in your fitness and overall health?

What do you think you'd decide to do with your first million-dollar make?

What type of relationship do you hope to establish?

What good deeds do you would like to accomplish?

What is a new dish you would want to explore?

What book new would you want to go through?

What book, article or music would you like to see published?

Exercise #5

Make a list of your achievements and create your personal eulogy. It's true that no one wants to think about their death however, we all end up dying at some moment in time. The point in this practice is to visualize the end you want to reach. It is not my intention to think about what you've accomplished through your entire life. In this particular exercise, consider what you'd like other people to think about you. What do you wish that others have to say about you? What would you like to be remembered for? What would you have wanted to achieve prior to that day? What do you hope to accomplish? affect the lives of others? What kind of job or service do you want to pursue, when it's relevant? This activity will provide some clues about what you can turn into goals.

Exercise #6

Make vision boards. If you're not aware what a vision board actually is, it's an assortment of pictures and words that express your hopes and desires. It lets you know what things you love and that will bring you joy. Remember the days of elementary school, when you'd cut and paste pictures on construction paper. When you do it when you are an adult it's known as the vision board. It's fun to complete this exercise using images from old magazines, however you can also make one on the internet. Once you have completed creating your dream board you can post it somewhere you can view it each day.

Exercise #7

Activism. There are clues in feelings that make you feel either positive or negatively. Examine the actions or injustices that you feel triggers more than you normally. What limitation or disability have you overcome? What is it that you are angry about? What people do you most compassionate towards? What can you learn from your experience?

Exercise #8 - Create Life Vision Statements

Utilizing the information you learned from the previous exercises, make the life-vision statements. The life-vision statement should be an ideal description of the ideal, desirable state of mind. Visions should not just be created in your mind however, it must be written down and graphically depicted. In this task, you'll create a vision statement that addresses 10 important areas of your life: spiritual, health personal growth, partner/spouse as well as family and friends financial, career and recreation, living space and community. Begin by defining or revising what success means in each of these areas. It's helpful to close your eyes during this exercise in order to reconnect with your soul and your true self since your real self lies within. Let go of any negative or painful thoughts that are trying to change your goals. It is important to remember that those difficult experiences should show your ability to overcome and not limit your thoughts. If you've been through the effects of abuse and other major failures in your life, then you will be able to conquer the minor issues like boredom, drifting working too much, and so on. Take a look at the examples provided from the following table to assist you write down your vision statements.

While you write your statement of your vision, you can begin to visualize yourself in the perfect state, possessing everything that you wrote down. It is crucial to transform the statements into pictures and feelings of euphoria. However you'll discover where you are in the middle and that's the reason why you should be pursuing your ambitions. Ideally, you must have goals for every aspect of your life, and want to create the life that is in alignment with your mission goals. You don't need to take on them at once however, understanding them will aid in defining your life's strategy.

In short it is important to brainstorm, think about the legacy goals, defining success, making an outline of your vision and creating vision statements are your most important steps to lay the basis for your goals. Be committed to this task prior to moving onto the next step. You will likely have to complete this discovery work. You've not responded to these questions and, actually, you've been avoiding them as nobody has committed you to doing this. No teacher, parent or pastor will ever insist on this from you. It is something that you must take on for yourself. This is the reason it's likely to require mental strength to deal with the challenges of this sort and is one of the primary reasons why people are stuck. It is a process of spiritual exploration that can be emotionally charged or even frightening. It is similar to taking medicine. It is difficult but beneficial, so take the time to do the exercises.

If you're not able to do the exercises, make sure to read the story from the intro to make sure you know where you're likely to end up if you fail to complete this section. The planning phase is vitally important. If you don't take the effort to make this decision, you'll not be at your potential and it's unlikely you'll sustain the success you have achieved. If you require help in the exercise, think about finding an accountability partner, or group of people to tackle the exercises together.

For those who have not completed these exercises would be the official end of the book, as the rest of the book will build upon the outcomes of the planning stage. I hope you'll come back to finish these exercises soon, when you realize that this fundamental work is essential. For those who have completed these exercise of planning, congratulations! you're well-prepared to take your next step.

Presto!

Vision statements and dreams throughout your life

Step 2 - Analyze Step 2 - Make Goals that are SMART.

After you've completed the planning stage to establish your goals and have a better understanding of your ideal life, it's time to conduct some research. What do you hope to accomplish in the wake of the research? Let's look at what you've put down. Consider the vision lists, statements, as well as all the clues and ah-ha revelations you have discovered and convert the lists into S.M.A.R.T. goals. It is

160

an acronym that identifies the five main features of a legitimate goal. The following explains the definition of SMART goals, and how exactly to develop them:

S- Specific

Is your goal specific? The goals you set should be clearly clear and unambiguous. The more precise the objective, the easier for you to know when you reach it. It is recommended to have at the very least one goal for every major area of your life, which you can define during your planning stage. Take a look at both short-term and long-term about the types of goals you would like to accomplish. Review the vision statements and consider the accomplishments that will help bring these goals to fruition.

Vision statement: It's essential for myself to live in a close-knit family. I want my kids to develop an enduring sense of family history and strong bonds with their aunts, grandparents uncles, cousins, and aunts.

The weakest goal I have is that it is to spend more time with my family.

Particular Goals: My aim is to host and/or initiate games nights with my family.

M Measurable

How can you gauge your improvement? What is more what will you know when you're completed? You must include physical attributes such as "how numerous" and "how much" when stating your objective. For instance, if you're looking savings, write the amount you intend to save, either in increments or in a certain amount, or by a certain period of time. This will be simpler to monitor and improve the likelihood of success. Simply saying you want to save money at the end of the year isn't enough However, stating that you're aiming to save each week $20 or $200 by December is a more accurate measurement. Furthermore, it can be encouraging to see tangible indicators of your goal as you progress. This means you will be able to acknowledge the accomplishments you make instead of focusing on the times that you don't adhere to your plan. Other measurement types are common like count, volume or amount of times, rate of the timer, percent trend, etc. .... It is generally better to stick with objective measures like those listed above rather than subjective ones that can be dependent on judgement and interpretation. For instance, to show the number of times you're planning to perform something, you can use numbers instead of using words like several, frequently never, frequently, or even numerous.

The weakest goal I have is that it is spend quality time with my loved ones regularly.

A Measurable Objective: My aim is to host events for my family three times during this year. By listing that you will host three events, you have established an measurable number; if you host four events you'll be over your goal and if you have only two events, you'll be short of your target. Your measurement will give you a target to aim to. In this case it is possible to start to pencil in the three occasions you'll hold on a calendar and then you'd put a huge green check-mark for the day you get to spend the most time together with family.

A- Attainable

Is your goal attainable? That is your goal must be achievable. You must have the capacity or the talent to accomplish it, or acquire the necessary skills. The goals may be difficult and require commitment or sacrifice however, they should be feasible, even slightly possible. Are you in a position to achieve it? Or can you be taught to do it? If you've always dreamed of playing basketball with the NBA and you're now aged 48 and haven't played before, I'd say it's impossible and completely impossible. If you'd like to be athletically healthy enough to participate within a regional league it could be possible.

Our Goal: My goal is to travel to all states within 48 days.

Attainable Goals: My goal is to travel to California and Nevada in the summer break this year.

Relevant

Is your goal relevant? This means that your goal must be essential to you. The majority of the work involved in determining the things that matter to you was completed in the initial planning phase which is why you're going over that information once more. Deciding whether a goal's important or not is closely tied to your desire and determination. If, for instance, you're aiming to become an NBA player however you aren't one exercising and aren't willing to put in the effort, then becoming an NBA player isn't your primary goal. It is possible that you have the capability to do it, and you may even be thinking about it as a means of achieving achieve a goal however, your motivation is a sign of the value you put on the idea. It is essential to be transparent with yourself regarding what you're willing take on when deciding on your target. This is a different approach that you were using in the planning stage. This is a shift into an attitude of commitment that will make your goal more relevant. That's why goals are actually your contractual agreement with your self. If you're not ready to enter into a binding agreement with yourself for the achievement of your goal the goal is merely an idea or a dream and not a goal at least not right now. One of the worst things you could do is be a lie to yourself and create an objective which you aren't planning to work hard to make it occur. You must be true to yourself and concentrate on what you would like to achieve in your life. If you do not meet your goals in this aspect It is very likely that you'll spend much time pursuing the aim and won't achieve it even if you achieve it.

Aimless Goal: Though I don't cook as often I'm planning to go to culinary school and become a chef just like my friend who makes lots of money from it.

Relevant Goal: I have always enjoyed baking, and it feels special when I get to serve and entertain people. I'll learn how to perfect this key lime recipe, and then enter into two different contests. in the end, I'll be able to transform this into a lucrative revenue stream.

T- Time-Bound

Is your goal timely? Also do you have time periods, dates for milestones or a deadline? The time component is what defines the date of completion of the objective. What date do you anticipate to be able to complete this goal? It is helpful to set both long-term and short-term objectives. At the end of the process you'll break your goals down into specific actions you'll need to accomplish within that timeframe. These tasks will also include an element of time. If you don't set time limitations then you risk of taking a long time or not being able to complete. You must be realistic about the time you set to complete your goal. At while you also would like to be a more aggressive to create the impression of urgency.

My weak goal: I'll bake key lime pie this year.

Time-Bound Goal: I'll bake key lime pie to bake to be used in the bake-off competition at church in September, and for the Christmas party at work in December.

Setting goals and making them SMART goals can be difficult for many to comprehend at first. Each goal must meet the criteria of all five. If this is all new to you, don't be discouraged if you can not get it right because it requires time and practice. People tend to ignore the measurable component or overlook the realizable element of their goal, therefore, check your goals again to make sure the five elements are in place. If all five elements are in place, the likelihood to accomplish your goal rises dramatically. If you need additional help, email coachclaudette@youworktoomuch.com to get additional assistance.

Exercise #9

Try to turn your visions into realistic goals. Each section should at the very least be able to accomplish one target, but you should create as many goals possible goals. Make sure to list as many of them as possible. If you look at this in terms of the main life categories, you will be creating a sense of balance rather than focusing only on the area that causes you the most suffering. Check out an example in the table below.

Exercise #10

There will be a mixed assortment of goals. Some are related to performance as well as new skills or habit-forming. The goal should be labeled according to the date of completion you want to achieve it in terms of the short term (less than 6 months) or intermediate (6 to 24 months) and longer-term (greater that 24 months). It is important to include goals that are long-term because they need to be addressed a bit at each time, and can assist you in making better choices about what you will spend your energy on in the short-term. Understanding what you'd like to achieve in the long run will allow you avoid things which aren't aligned with your goals that you've determined with a lot of effort. In addition, goals that are long-term tend to feel more satisfying due to the effort and discipline they require to reach them. Check out the some examples below in table.

Ideally, you've set a variety of goals by now. Do you realize how linking your goals to your goals and vision statements, and making them smart goals will ensure that you have a well-balanced approach to life? You will have a clearer idea of what you would like to achieve, the reason, and when. If you've completed the Analytic Exercises, great job! You are now about halfway through the entire process.

Chapter 9: Understanding The Dynamics Of Workaholism

Do you feel an overwhelming need to be productive all day long? Do you carry your work everywhere, regardless of where you are even by your bedside prior to going to bed? Do you experience a feeling of guilt or regret whenever you are doing nothing and feel like it's impossible to leave without a job to complete? Do you feel like you are working too hard and at the expense of your family and your personal satisfaction?

If you responded yes to one or more of the questions above it is possible that you are showing symptoms of an the signs of addiction to work or alcoholism.

Like other types of addiction, workaholism can be defined by a range of distinct signs. One of them is an unsettling sense of satisfaction by working for hours on end. It is precisely this feeling of satisfaction that prevents workaholics from changing their working habits.

Addiction to work

However, in contrast to addiction to drugs where the addiction takes the form from an outside object (i.e. alcohol and drugs) working-related addictions are an addiction that is associated with an intangible thing, that is, work.

In reality, the concept of work isn't considered to be in the eyes of society as morally unsound or unethical. It's actually something that every responsible person to be involved in. Why is it that workaholism is thought to be unhealthful?

The issue with workaholism lies from the inability of a person to disconnect from work until exhaustion. For those who are addicted to work, nothing less than fatigue that is the natural result of excessive work can stop them from what they're doing. It's a type of disordered behavior that is characterized by an inability to distinguish between work and private life.

If it is not controlled, workaholism can cause a variety of negative consequences. In the long-term the effects could affect the overall physical, emotional well-being, as well as mental.

Workaholism and its effects

The most obvious and visible results of being a working-aholic can be observed in one's physical appearance. Constantly exposing the body to stress by sleeping infrequently even if they do, and not exercising regularly causes damage and wear. Numerous studies have revealed the negative consequences of stress, which include the formation of gastrointestinal and cardiovascular diseases, diminished stamina as well as the diminution of our immune system of the body, among other things.

Stress can also cause lack of focus and concentration. The ability to focus and concentrate is linked with an energized body, which means that a body constantly stressed out is harder than normal for your brain concentrate. This becomes more obvious when you don't take the opportunity to have a break.

In the same way, the negative consequences of working only to the individual suffering of it but to those who are around them. Because a significant portion of the time a person with a job is devoted to the work he or she is doing so they are only able to spend a few minutes or even time to build positive relationships with others. In general, relationships require time and in the absence of this condition makes these relationships weak even if they are not completely sustainable.

In light of all these negative outcomes the question that needs for an immediate response is how did workaholism develop? Certain researchers suggest that the addiction to alcohol and drugs could have a genetic component, which means that the susceptibility to these forms of addiction is traceable to the ancestors of one's. Is the same for those who work? What triggers can trigger this kind of bizarre behavior?

Identifying the Triggers for Workaholism

On the surface it could appear to be an inherent tendency to work longer hours than is normal. In an environment that puts the importance of dedication and sacrifice in pursuit of objectives in the workplace, a person who is a workaholic represents the selfless, hardworking worker -- the type of person other people must admire and imitate.

There is something that is twisted about the notion of workaholism being the ideal way of life. Because, being a worker is anything not the ideal. While it isn't a reflection of the way professionals should conduct their careers Being a workaholic is a type of obsessional behavior disorder that is the result of many triggers, none of which is positive.

Here are a few of the most frequent triggers for alcohol dependence:

Deep-seated anxieties

People with insecurities tend to make excuses for other things to cover up the things that they are unsure about. For those who are people who work hard, their desire to put in long hours until exhaustion reflects an insatiable desire or a desire to prove themselves to other people. They are buried under many layers of obligations to prove they're capable. They fool themselves into thinking they're confident in their self-esteem and worth even when they're not.

Tendencies for escapism

Escapism refers to the strong, almost irresistible need to run as far as you can from an issue or issue. For those who are a workaholic, the escape takes the shape of work. They can find the refuge they need in their work, even if their jobs begin to impact their mental and physical health in part because they prefer to endure the stress of work instead of face their other problems confronting them head-on.

A misplaced sense of perfection

A large portion of people adhere to an extremely high standard on the way they perform their responsibilities and duties. Although this isn't necessarily a negative thing but it does cause a situation in which the standard they set is not sustainable in the end. A quest for perfection only creates a flood of despair and delusion since it will never be attained no matter how much you try to achieve it. For those who are a workaholic, this results in an obsession with goals that ultimately results in nothing.

Incredibility in the capabilities of other people

A close relationship to perfectionionism and perfectionists is the inability to have belief in the abilities of others. The people who work hard do it because they believe that in their own way, no other person can do the job better than they do. In the end, they assume all responsibility for themselves, having a monopoly on tasks in the fear that delegating these tasks to other people will cause a lower output.
Unfounded fears
In these days, it's difficult to not be worried about the prospects for one's career. With unemployment rates in the midst of a new record, and numerous companies embarking on mass reductions in staff, it's obvious why there are a few people who are worried about losing their jobs push them to take on more. For them

they are able to count on their jobs to mean much, particularly when losing their jobs mean the inability to cover loans for cars, mortgages, home rentals, college loans as well as utility bills, among other essential costs. If working all day long late into the night, and retaining these jobs, being a complete workaholic is only a consequence of their current circumstances.

The causes of workaholism do not only include those mentioned within this section. In reality, there are a variety of other causes which can trigger an increase in this mental disorder. It is essential that triggers are identified because the first step in fighting workaholism is identification of the problems that cause this problems. To support this, the next chapter provides information about the necessity to take concrete steps towards reducing but not entirely the workaholic habits.

Implementing Concrete Steps to Stop the stigma of being a Workaholic

Due to the complex nature of the different triggers that lead to the condition, it's clear that getting rid of this problem is not likely to be a simple task. It is evident that many adjustments will need to be made during the process. As is discussed in following chapters the process of getting rid of this type of addiction isn't something that can be accomplished in a single day. Similar to any other disorder of the same kind recovery requires a great deal of commitment, dedication and discipline as well as the determination to improve your life.

The process of healing should begin by recognizing the issue. In this instance the issue is the desire to devote an extended amount of time doing work that is detrimental to the other aspects of the life of a person. It is crucial to recognize this as without it there will be no clear ways to deal with it.

Priorities to be assessed

Start by reviewing your priorities. For those who are a workaholic, their primary priority set on their job. To correct the situation, this priority should be adjusted to allow for other items in your life.

Therefore you should take a long, thorough look at the things or people you cherish the most and assess their importance. Determine what or who deserves the highest attention from you and then make any necessary adjustments from there. The following are typically at the top of everyone's priority list:

* Family, which comprises immediate relatives, spouses and children;

* health or the absence any serious illness or at a minimum an effective treatment of the physical condition of one's self;

* Personal happiness and emotional well-being.

* Money and everything it buys.

The most important thing is to understand that, beyond your professional life There are other aspects in your life that need to be given more weight. It is your responsibility to determine what those aspects are.

The huge image

To understand the dangers of being too busy at work, it is important to place things in the proper setting. Take a look at the bigger image. Every time you go to bed for an entire night in bed to complete an assignment, you should give an answer to these questions: Does this task truly require a an unavoidable urgency? Do you know how to accomplish this without jeopardizing your personal life and relations with other people especially your family? What are the consequences of completing this project likely to impact your life? Are you simply assuming the responsibility of a job that was supposed to be performed by others?

It is crucial to stress that the purpose here is not to provide an excuse to not work. It's not the case at all. The ability to see the bigger image is essential for those who work hard but fail to place their actions in the context of their actions. The tendency to work, work and then work more leads to their inability to discern the right and wrong actions to take. not be doing.

In gaining a macro view of what is happening, people who work hard should be able to be aware of the effects of their commitment to work with regard to their personal lives and also their family.

Conclusion

Being afflicted by anxiety and addiction to alcohol at simultaneously is an enormous challenge. If you're reading this book to help someone you love Do them a favor and attempt to understand the reasons they're suffering and put you in their position to ensure you can understand them better.

People who are suffering from anxiety and working-related stress are amazing people inside. Give them the opportunity to demonstrate that , and help them get rid of the fog created by their condition. Keep in mind that they didn't have a choice to be as they are. It just happens that working-out is the only option they have to prevent their excessive anxiety attack.

If, on the other hand you're here because you're suffering from it and want to treat it, I'd like you to be aware of these words: The sole moment when a problem becomes unsolvable is when you let it occur. No matter what other people might tell you to discourage yourself. They don't know what you're talking about and you know what's the best for you. Nobody else has that knowledge than you. If you really desire to get rid of your disease begin by forming your mind to create your own life. Whatever other people say, it will not occur unless you decide to and then actually do it.

www.ingramcontent.com/pod-product-compliance
Lightning Source LLC
Chambersburg PA
CBHW060332030426
42336CB00011B/1308